# PARALLEL WORLDS

# PARALLEL WORLDS

## A Mother's Journey through a Son's Addiction

### KATHLEEN ARCH

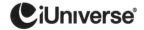

PARALLEL WORLDS
A MOTHER'S JOURNEY THROUGH A SON'S ADDICTION

iUniverse books may be ordered through booksellers or by contacting:

iUniverse
1663 Liberty Drive
Bloomington, IN 47403
www.iuniverse.com
1-800-Authors (1-800-288-4677)

Because of the dynamic nature of the Internet, any web addresses or links contained in this book may have changed since publication and may no longer be valid. The views expressed in this work are solely those of the author and do not necessarily reflect the views of the publisher, and the publisher hereby disclaims any responsibility for them.

Any people depicted in stock imagery provided by Thinkstock are models, and such images are being used for illustrative purposes only.
Certain stock imagery © Thinkstock.

ISBN: 978-1-4917-5942-4 (sc)
ISBN: 978-1-4917-5943-1 (hc)
ISBN: 978-1-4917-5941-7 (e)

Library of Congress Control Number: 2015903387

Print information available on the last page.

iUniverse rev. date: 03/17/2015

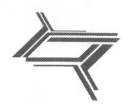

# CONTENTS

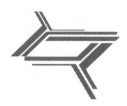

# INTRODUCTION

This is the story of my son's battle with the disease of addiction and the resulting effects on our entire family. Some of the passages in these first chapters are taken from the journal I wrote during this difficult time.

The middle section of this book is dedicated to the stories of those around me—stories of hope, stories of loss, and stories of pain and struggles. Some stories were written by survivors, and some were submitted by a loved one who tells the story of a soul gone too soon.

Please tread softly as you embrace the sentiment behind the struggle. In sharing our stories, though often difficult to put into words, we offer a personal insight into the world of addiction. We help each other when we offer our experiences. The more we speak out about the disease of addiction, the greater is the chance to prevent the spread of the stigma associated with the disease.

In the final chapter of *Parallel Worlds*, you are invited to add your own messages of hope within the blank spaces intended for your thoughts. Perhaps you will find a way to reach your inner soul by expressing your emotions in the "Meditative Journey" section of this book.

Addiction … a disease of addiction … the mere thought of addiction—it is a journey never imagined by a parent, a family member, or a friend of someone caught in its destructive web. We know we can control addiction, but if we end the stigma associated with this terrible disease, perhaps we can help prevent it.

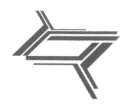

# IN THE BEGINNING

Today, I am a stranger in a strange new world but not the world to which I was born. I do not recognize this strange new world; I did not ask to be part of this strange new world. Sadly, here I am—unsettled, unsure of my next step, and drowning in the uncertainty this new world represents.

How did I come to be part of this world? To understand it, one would have to experience the beginning, the middle, and perhaps the end, although the end has not been clearly defined yet. The beginning was simple; I was unaware of the possibility that a parallel world could exist. Like many before me, I naively was forced into this new world by a series of events. Those events, which unfolded over fifteen hundred days ago, opened Pandora's box.

Pandora's box is an artifact in Greek mythology, but today, "opening Pandora's box" refers to an action that may seem small or innocent but results in severe and far-reaching consequences.

The Pandora's box that was opened, which led me into this strange new world, is called addiction. *Addiction*—it deserves very little respect, but unfortunately, it takes center stage, at least until it can be stopped or upstaged by a power greater than its force. Addiction—sadly but quite often—will win the battle it enters. Addiction cares not for the casualties it leaves behind—the human souls dissolved into an abyss (regions of Hell conceived to be a bottomless pit). Far too many have joined me in this strange new world, and far too many continue to line up behind me and watch, powerlessly, as their lives unfold into Satan's world of addiction.

My son did not go willingly into the world of addiction; he had help—someone posing as a friend held open the door and beckoned him into this strange new world. Like many, my son was drawn by the power of the promise of relief from his undiagnosed depression. Like so many before him, he was offered a resting place for his mind, and he gladly signed on. He believed that he would be able to clear his mind, and he then would come back to the world to which he was born. But this experiment failed—a failure beyond his wildest imagination—and it opened Pandora's box, which led me to join him in this strange new world.

I have no idea where this world will lead us, but for today, the power and the force of addiction have yet again destroyed my child. In turn, addiction has consumed me and taken away my ability to see a brighter tomorrow for either of us. It appears that the power of the addiction grows stronger with each passing day, and I grow weaker as the day fades into the night. Today, I am left with only a shadow of the child I brought into this world—the stronger the pull, the stranger the world and the deeper the abyss.

To wish for a brighter tomorrow for my son is to wish that his journey had not taken place, but it did. To wish that I knew what tomorrow might bring would mean this strange new world was a nightmare from which I would emerge, but sadly, it is my new world, and it is real.

Today, in this moment in time, I am but a stranger in a strange new world. Please, do not follow me.

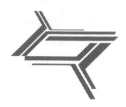

# I CANNOT TELL YOU

*A mother's struggle with a son's addiction*

It has been just over four years, and I cannot tell you how I feel. I cannot tell you that I am terrified, every day that you will be gone tomorrow. I cannot take the chance that what I say today will cause you to step back into the nightmare of your old ways. I cannot tell you that I still cry myself to sleep at night, because I fear you will be gone when I awake. I cannot tell you that not a day goes by without visions of your past haunting my daily life. I cannot tell you that every time I hug you, I squeeze a little tighter, as I fear it may be the last time I embrace you. I cannot tell you any of this, because these things are my issues; they are my fears.

Your road has been bumpy and stressful, and it has come with many setbacks, yet you are here today, stronger, wiser, and more determined than ever to win your battle with addiction. I am so proud of you for your ability to see beyond your past and for taking the steps necessary to rebuild your life. I, however, am stuck in my nightmare, and I must find my way out.

With each passing day, I pray that time will heal the wounds your lifestyle created. I know you are becoming stronger, but somehow, I have grown weaker in my ability to see beyond your past.

As a mother, it is my job to protect you—at least it was while you were young and inexperienced. As a mother, it is my job to see you through the challenges of growing up. As a mother, however, I have no turn-off button that allows me to walk away or to look the other way. I cannot forget the things that matter, nor can I filter out yesterday's memories or tomorrow's nightmares.

Support groups encourage us to "stop, let it be, move on with your life, and learn to be happy again." What they do not understand is this: you are part of my life. You are part of my happy, and you are part of my soul. Therefore, I cannot tell you how I feel today, but perhaps tomorrow will bring a sense of closure. Perhaps tomorrow, we will both be strong enough to face the pain that yesterday's lifestyle has caused. Perhaps!

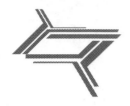

# Don't Mind Me; I'm Just Buffering

Have you ever downloaded a song on your computer or waited for a web page to open? If so, you know only too well what the spinning circle in the middle of the screen represents—your computer is buffering. The page or the song is waiting to open, and your life is on hold.

Today, I am buffering. Today, I am taking a moment to digest the events of the last four days, and today, I am slowly returning to my life.

Like so many parents of an addicted child, my life is on pause. My son, now twenty-four years old, is back in a treatment program after nearly two years of being "clean." The events that unfolded are part of the nightmare of addiction—a nightmare experienced by far too many parents, normal people from all walks of life.

I saw the signs—I know the signs only too well—and I started to do what every parent of an addict does: I put a plan in motion.

For me, the signs are the little things; things that most people might ignore. My son loves to write; he writes songs and letters and writes as a way to journal his thoughts. When he is heading back down the slippery slope of addiction, however, his writing style changes. His words begin to slant in the opposite position, literally.

He switches back and forth between printing and cursive, his penmanship is impeccable in the beginning but becomes barely legible as he continues to write. Little pictures are drawn in the corners of the paper; video games are designed in great detail—each one unrelated to the other but all residing together on the same page. No blank space is left on the paper; every square inch is covered with words, drawings, and strange symbols. This is how I know that something's up! Something is happening, and I need to step back into the picture.

As parents, we know our children's habits all too well, but even when we recognize the signs, it can be heartbreaking to see it coming, again. My son disappeared for hours—no phone call, no text message, no response. When something like this happens to a parent, panic starts. Tears cloud your eyes, and your heart beats so fast that you can hardly breathe. You know only too well what's coming next, and what is about to happen; again … relapse!

For me, however, this time was different. This time, it came out of the blue, and this time it scared me more than ever before. Why was this time different? Because the last text message from my son, I received four hours earlier that day, said, "I'm done, Mama. I don't want this life anymore, and I can't stop it from happening. Nobody understands me; nobody can help me this time …, *and I don't want to do this life anymore. I love you* Mama Bear, but I am done." For me, the "Mama Bear" was the clincher. He usually says "Mama Bear" when he is in a "great" mood, or when he is uncontrollably sad and deeply depressed. So this time was different, and this time, I needed a new plan—and I needed it fast.

I reached out to a select few people via private message on Facebook— those I felt would really listen and perhaps have an idea I had yet to try. It worked! I was showered with support, all with one response in common: "What can I do to help?" At this point, I could no longer control the tears. How was it possible that so many wonderful parents could relate to my situation? And how sad that they could.

Most of us have special people in our lives to whom we turn in our time of need, but when addiction is on the table, that time of need is very different. When addiction is running the show, the possibility of death stares you in the face. Addiction is just waiting to have the final word.

Over the next several days, messages from complete strangers poured in, at twelve o'clock, one o'clock and even two o'clock in the morning, all asking the same questions: "Has he called you yet? Is he okay? Are you okay?" I knew some of the people who responded by name, but some messages were from people I had never met—messages from complete strangers who somehow learned a parent was in trouble. They did what all parents of an addicted child do in such a situation; they stepped in simply because they cared.

For me, this story continues, and as of this today, my son is back in treatment. But for many other parents, their story had a much different ending. So here is my question: what can we do that has not yet been tried? What can we do to give back to those who step in when our loved one is in trouble? Do we give back, and do we pay it forward?

We do what we can to provide support to parents in need. We provide education; we host a support group; we hold panel-group discussions; and we offer our hearts. Personally, I journal my story, and I host support meetings when I can.

For today, I am still buffering as I try to return to a semi-normal day, and I pray that treatment works—this time. I pray that the knight in shining armor who came to rescue my son knows that I can never say thank you enough times for saving my child's life. But I can also pay it forward by continuing to do what I do. I write, and I journal my experiences with the hope that what I write will somehow offer strength to another parent in need of support.

Sometimes buffering is all that we can do until we find the strength to breathe again. Then we smile and say, "How can I help you?"

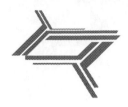

# Just Show Me

Today has been a bit of a challenge, though I don't know why. I heard a song on the radio by Joan Baez, "There but for Fortune," and I cried. I am not sure what brought it on, but then again … I guess I do. Maybe it's the past five months—during which I hoped to move but it continued to fall apart—that has brought me to this place. Maybe it's the actual move that finally took place and the exhaustion that followed. Or maybe it's just the life of the mother of a child suffering the disease of addiction.

The words of the song that registered most with me are these:
*Show me the prison, show me the jail*
*Show me the prisoner, whose life has gone stale*

This life, the life of an addict is you or me; it is anyone, at any time, in any place. There are many reasons why, yet there is not a reason in the world why this should happen to any of our children. "Show me the prisoner, whose life has gone stale"—those words keep me engaged in the struggle and involved in my child's life as an addict. His life has gone stale, and I am now a prisoner in a world that does not get noticed.

Over the past few days, something has changed yet again. The glimmer in my child's eyes has once again disappeared. The fear of relapse, the fear of jail, and the ultimate fear of loss of life has gripped my soul. I cannot shake the terrible feeling that the worst is yet to come. Can any parent of an addict shake that fear? Are we destined to a life of fear? Perhaps.

I don't have my answers, so I don't have your answers either. All I have is a gut feeling that only a parent of an addict can understand. Addiction can and often does, sit dormant for months or even years, but that fear—the fear only a parent can realize—never sits dormant. It always rides too close to the surface. Perhaps in some sadistic way, it is preparing us for the inevitable.

My son is different today than he was yesterday. There is something building up inside him. I've seen the signs before and, just as in the past; I am powerless to stop him. I can only do what so many before me have done: *watch*. I can see what many others before me have seen—the torture of the addiction slowing becoming powerful once again.

So for today, I ask him, "What's happening, sweet boy?" Can I stop it? Can I help him? I ask him once again, "Please, sweet child of mine, just show me; just tell me how I can help you." But there is only sadness in his eyes.

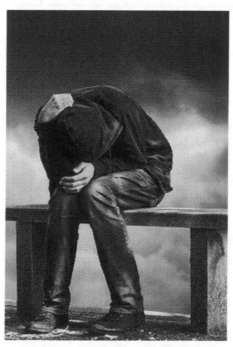

*For many, this is the picture of a homeless drug addict.*
*But for someone, this is a picture of a beloved son they could not help*

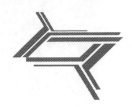

# IN MY OPINION

It has been 1,445 days since addiction entered my life. It has been 1,445 days since addiction took over my child's life. And it has taken me 1,445 days to come to grips with what addiction has done to our lives, but so far, by the grace of God, we have survived.

In my opinion, this new life—the life addiction brought to the table—was not caused by my son's inability to say no. It is my opinion that none of our children willingly woke up one day and said, "Addiction, please come entertain me and transform me," or "Addiction, please take my life."

My life was simple 1,446 days ago—neatly displayed on the mantel like a trophy. My vision for my son, 1,446 days ago, was rather simple—college, which was going well; marriage, perhaps part of my child's future; and grandchildren, perhaps one day blessing his life and mine. It is my opinion that 1,446 days ago, my life—and his—was on track.

Today, 1,445 days later, I firmly believe we are still on track but with a far different plan. Of this new plan that the universe has in store for us—and for any parent of an addict—I have no opinion. But I can tell you, without a shadow of a doubt, that addiction has the strongest pull and the most substantial influence known to man. I do have a strong opinion that there was nothing I could have done that would have changed what addiction has done to our lives. We are powerless to change that which we do not see coming.

I recently overheard a conversation between two moms. One asked the other, "Do you still love your child the same, now that he is an addict?" I stood frozen as I watched this exchange. It felt like an eternity before the mother of the addicted child finally responded, "Do I still love my child the same? Why would I love him less? He is still my child. Would you have asked that question if my child had been diagnosed with cancer?" As the two women parted, tears rolled down my face. I realized that many parents walk this same path with a child struggling with addiction. Many parents are surrounded by the same ignorance—the ignorance that produces the stigma associated with the disease of addiction.

It is my opinion that most of mankind is made up of kind and caring individuals. Addiction has no prerequisite, just as ignorance has no prerequisite. Anyone is invited to join the club. Addiction cares not if you are black or white. Addiction cares not if you are rich or poor, popular or awkward. Addiction cares not if you are a respected young athlete or a science "nerd." Ignorance, in my opinion, has the same qualifications; we just never expect such actions to come from our family or close circle of friends.

"Do you love your child the same, now that he is an addict?" This question hurts my heart. But I think what bothered me most when I heard that question was the look on the face of the mother whose child suffers from the disease of addiction. The look was not one of shock but of sheer pain. That look told me that this was not the first time such a hurtful question had been asked.

Addiction is a disease. Addiction is like a cancer that grows within our loved ones, our precious children. Addiction is like a tumor that cannot be removed. Addiction is a condition that may go into remission, but it can also resurface at any time. Addiction is a disease with no cure—but it can be successfully treated. Addiction is a disease that destroys the entire family, and addiction, like cancer, can be fatal.

It is my opinion that we still have a very long way to go before addiction will be viewed with the same respect as other diseases. We still have a very long way to go before we find a cure for the disease of ignorance. Would I rather my child suffer the disease of ignorance than the disease of addiction? That is a tough question, as both diseases destroy families and friendships. Ignorance has a higher rate of survival, perhaps that's because it has so many willing participants. Nobody wants to be an addict, but it seems that many enjoy the role of ignorance.

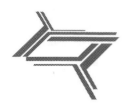

# ONE GIANT PUZZLE

L ife is a giant puzzle, and the pieces seldom fit. I never thought I'd be faced with the need to make so many profound decisions that so greatly affect those I love. While my tasks are small when I compare them to those in my current circle of friends, I realize that all difficult decisions are simply that—difficult decisions.

I have friends who have faced struggles far greater than my own, yet they are here for me as if to say, my struggles somehow compare in magnitude to their struggles. Never underestimate the power of support, no matter where it comes from. Support is all around us. Sadly, many continue to struggle alone—in isolation and in fear of the unknown.

When we deal with addiction in a loved one, we struggle alone. Some people may take up jogging, some may take up yoga, and many simply smile and walk away, and struggle alone. I have done all of the above, and I have no idea what truly works and what does not. We are in the same boat, yet struggle alone.

My son has an unbearable struggle in life; the disease of addiction is his Achilles' heel. Do you remember the story of Achilles? In Greek mythology, when Achilles was a baby, it was foretold that he would die young. To prevent his death, his mother, Thetis, took Achilles to the River Styx, which was supposed to offer powers of invulnerability. There, she dipped his body into the water. But as Thetis held Achilles by the heel, his heel was not washed over by the water of the magical river. Achilles grew up to be a man of war who survived many great battles. But one day, a poisonous arrow was shot at him and lodged in his heel, killing him shortly thereafter.

As parents, we try to protect our children from the many evils that prevail in life. We try to navigate them in the direction of hope for a great future, and we try to offer alternative lifestyles, should addiction grab them. I sent my son to some of the best rehab centers that I could afford. I drove him to support meetings, and I drove him to meet with great counselors, yet addiction is like a poisonous arrow lodged in his heel. Addiction will often win the battle, but I fight daily not to allow addiction to win the war.

Today, again I can say my son is clean—but I cannot say, with any great authority, that he will remain clean. I can say that today he is working his program, and today he is focused. I can say that today I am breathing in and breathing out without the same degree of fear that crippled my days in the past. But I also can tell you that today is only the beginning of a very long road—a road that I am willing to face head-on, alongside my child.

My dream for every person who reads my story is to find peace of mind. We are working hard toward better education. We are working hard to find greater solutions and better ways to prevent the tragic loss of one more innocent life to the disease of addiction.

Always remember: we are greater in strength when we are greater in number.

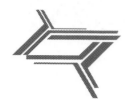

# If You're Reading
# This Letter

The story about John that you are about to read is real, though his name has been changed. In telling John's story, I hope that others who suffer the disease of addiction may find the strength to fight their demons and regain their sobriety.

At a recent support meeting, attended by those dealing with the drama of addiction, John caught my attention. He spoke with love in his heart, pain in his eyes, and conviction in his voice.

The following is John's story ...

> I have been addicted to many substances over many years, and I have tried to stop a number of times over the past ten years. I have hurt a great number of people in my life by the choices I have made. I have made amends for many of these choices, and I have fallen victim to these choices more times than I care to share. I asked to speak today to share with you the vision that changed my life.
>
> Approximately eighty-two days ago, I received a letter that was written to my mother nearly forty-four years ago by my father, who died in the Vietnam War in 1969. My mother carried this letter with her everywhere. I had never read the letter, nor had my mother ever shared with me my father's words. Every night, my mother would close her bedroom door and read my father's letter. Then she'd fall asleep, peacefully, with his memory tucked neatly under her pillow.

However, approximately eighty-two days ago, I received a package that contained two letters. One letter was marked "Read me first," and the other letter was worn and tattered, the ink on the envelope too faded to read. I opened the first letter; it was from my mother. I had not seen or spoken to my mother for many years, as my addiction had taken her place in my life. However, today my mother wrote:

My dear son,

I have loved you, and I have missed you terribly, but now I need you to listen as I tell you. You have been in my heart, in my soul, and in my thoughts every day of my life. While I understand it was your life choices that took you away, I know well that your heart and your love never left. I need to tell you something important, and I need you to hear my words and feel the emotion in my heart.

If you are reading this letter, it means I am no longer of this earth. I have known for several years that my health was failing but did not reach out to you, as I did not want to add to your burden. I know the disease of addiction has taken your body from me, but I also know your heart has never left, as I have felt you near me all the while.

I love you forever and always, and I will see you again one day in heaven—I will be standing beside your father to embrace you when you arrive. I will be smiling, and I will have my arms open wide, ready to hug you. However, my dear son, do not rush to see us, as we will wait an eternity; our hearts will never stray.

I do hope you find a way back to your life, and I hope you use your struggles to overcome addiction, as a way to help others in need. I do hope you know that I never stopped loving you. I was always there, in one fashion or another, when you felt alone or in need of love. I am always in your heart; you'll just need to listen a little harder now.

May you find some peace in knowing, how very much you have been loved.

With all my heart always,

Mom.

Those in attendance sat in silence. No one knew what to say or how to react. John reached into his pocket and pulled out the second letter. He shared only the first two paragraphs.

My dear Sara, the love of my life,

If you are reading this letter, it means I am no longer of this earth. However, I need to tell you something important. My heart will live on forever in the baby you are carrying, our son. I wish I were there to see his first smile and to hold him in my arms, but I know you will love him enough for the both of us. Sara, please name him John, after my father, the greatest man I ever knew. I know my father will protect him, just as I will protect him in spirit, until we are joined together in heaven.

Sara, please tell our son that there is nothing in this world he cannot accomplish if he wants it badly enough. Please tell him that I am proud of him and the man he is to become. Moreover, Sara, please tell him when the time comes, I will be waiting in heaven with a smile on my face and my arms open wide, ready to hug him for the first time. He is the product of our love, and he too will share this kind of love with his children, one day.

Love to both of you,

All my love, all my life,

Bill

John quietly folded the two letters and carefully placed them back in his pocket. With tears in his eyes, he continued. "I received both of these letters eighty-two days ago from a man with a big smile on his face and a warm glow about him. I was in a dark alley. I was hungry, I was cold, and I was wet from the rain. I was about to end my life, as I believed I had no way to regain my dignity. That was eighty-two days ago, and today, I am still here, and I am still clean."

John reached into his pocket for a third letter and said, "I wrote this letter to my mother, eighty-two days ago." Then he read, "Dear Mom, if you are reading this letter, it means I am no longer of this earth."

John put the third letter back in its envelope and placed it in his pocket with the other two letters. His voice was a whisper as he said, "As I was about to write the next line in my letter, a bright light caught my attention. A man appeared, as if out of nowhere, and handed me two letters. He whispered these words: 'Son, please do not finish your letter, for I need you to become the man I know you can become.'"

John then said, "Many will find my story to be nothing more than a drug-induced hallucination. But I believe this was my higher power reaching out to me, or perhaps it was the voice of my father."

As the meeting ended, tears fell, and the room was silent.

I share this story with you, as we all need to empathize and understand that it takes more strength to quit than it does to use drugs or alcohol. When fought alone, no war has a winner. It matters not what helps you to put down your drug of choice; it matters only that you do. Find your own higher power to help you move past your choices, before you write the words, "If you are reading this letter …"

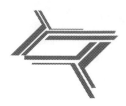

# I Will Not Tiptoe

Are you the parent of a child suffering the ill effects of addiction? Do you know someone who is suffering the ill effects of addiction?

In either case, you need to stand tall and not give in to the shame often associated with the ill effects of the disease of addiction.

We hide from that which we cannot bear. We hide from that which we do not understand. We hide from our family, from our friends, and sometimes, we hide from the person suffering the ill effects from the disease of addiction.

Such actions must not be confused with the notion that we are proud that a loved one is suffering the harmful effects of addiction. I am advocating, however, a community of our most cherished family and friends, in which we should not have to tiptoe around the subject of addiction. We should not be made to feel that something is terribly wrong in our parenting skills. We should not be made to feel alone, embarrassed, or ashamed of our child or loved one who is a victim of the disease of addiction.

We hide and isolate ourselves from those we love because society has not come to terms with the real measure of addiction. We see only what is most prominently displayed—the ugly non-truths about addiction. When a parent seeks help or asks for ideas or advice, they may need only for someone to listen. How sad that we, as a society, turn our heads and pretend not to hear the overwhelming panic, fear, and despair in the voice of a parent. We fail, as a society of intelligent people, when we judge that which we do not understand.

However, since I alone cannot end the misguided truth about the disease of addiction, I will continue to post comments on message boards and to write stories, with the hope of offering a resting place to someone in need. I believe that we show our greatest strength and compassion when we offer our love, unconditionally.

If you truly want to walk in the footsteps of a parent in need of help, I suggest that you attend a support meeting—sit quietly and just listen. Listen with your heart, not your mind. Listen, watch, and absorb the pain. You cannot judge that which you have not personally endured.

We are promoting better information, better education, and better resources. We are advocating legislature to catch up with and address the needs of those suffering the ill effects of addiction (medically and financially). We are helping the community in pain to find closure on a topic that seems to surface every time another child loses his or her battle with the disease of addiction. Why are we still walking through the Dark Ages or tiptoeing around the subject of addiction?

At a recent support meeting, a mother stood, her hands trembling as she spoke. "My sixteen-year-old son is battling addiction. At night when I tuck my younger children [ages nine and twelve] into bed, I gently whisper in their ears, 'I love you so much.' I tell them how much I value their existence, and I tell them how very proud I am of their daily choices. I do this nightly, with the hope that my gentle messages will be embedded in their minds. I do this to help shield them from the temptation of the cool-looking drug dealer, the one who patiently waits near the bus stop."

As she sat back in her chair, the room was silent. No one spoke, and the meeting adjourned. My heart hurt for her pain. My heart hurt, because I thoroughly understood her story.

I stopped tiptoeing 1,068 days ago, but I've yet to see much progress in our system. Change, education, compassion, and support for those in need—this is what I'm advocating. What are you doing to help those in need of support?

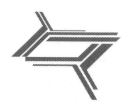

# WHY CAN'T I
# BELIEVE HIM?

Why is it so difficult to believe your child is clean when he or she tells you, "Mom stop, I'm clean." Why can't you stop obsessing about his or her addiction? Why can't you inhale and then exhale without feeling pain or fear?

When your child faces the disease of addiction, your life is forever changed. Why is it, when a friend tells you about the happy and fulfilling accomplishments of her child, and then she smiles and says, "So tell me—how is your child doing?" that you want to scream? You want to run away and pretend the woeful look on her face was meant for someone else. You need just *one* peaceful, enjoyable day without a single thought of addiction. Why is that so difficult to obtain?

My child has been clean (I believe) for nearly eighteen months, yet every time I see him, I am terrified he will be gone tomorrow. There are times when I go for days, for weeks, and even for months without the fear of losing him to an overdose. Still, I can't believe that he will be here tomorrow, let alone six months from now. I still have panic attacks when I hear of someone's child who is using. Am I fooling myself into believing that my child is clean and will remain clean?

Does this fear ever leave your side? Will the day ever come when you can look at your child with total comfort, knowing and believing that he has overcome his need to use—even when his disease of addiction is in remission?

Today was not a great day. Today, I saw my son as though I were first learning of his addiction, and today, I am withdrawing from life again. If this statement sounds familiar, then you need to understand that you are not alone in your struggles. You are not alone with your fears or frustrations. You are a parent in need of support. Support is greater some days and less comforting other days. You are a parent whose heart was filled with dreams of a brighter tomorrow, but at this very moment, you need to vent.

I wish I could tell you that tomorrow will bring closure, that this part of your life will eventually end, but I cannot tell you that. I cannot tell you that one day you will wake up and all your fears will be gone. I cannot tell you that there was a reason why all of this has happened to your child, to your family, and to your life.

What I can tell you, however, is that true support of family and friends will help. I can tell you that you will have days or perhaps weeks where your life will return to normal. And I can tell you that one day, you will be able to breathe without the fear that the other shoe is about to fall. I can tell you that for nearly every child who suffers the disease of addiction, treatment can work. I can tell you that the support that is waiting for you may help you to heal. There is no right or wrong way to deal with the drama that addiction has caused, but there is hope.

Support groups offer parents a place to vent, a place to cry, and a place to learn how to smile again. Support groups offer parents a place to feel normal in their suspicions, without the fear of being judged. Support groups provide a place to hear what other parents are doing to help regain their sanity.

I am lucky to have found my way to one such group, known as SOLACE—Surviving Our Loss with Awareness, Compassion and Empathy. This group was started by three incredible women, with the purpose of offering support for families who have lost a loved one to substance use and for families currently struggling with a loved one's addiction. SOLACE is my rock and my safe place to vent, to laugh, and to find my way back, each time I fall off the edge and fear the loss of my child. I encourage you to find a group to support your needs. Survival is easier when you have trusted people around you who understand your pain.

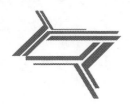

# TWO STEPS FORWARD, ONE STEP BACK

I got up today, and I smiled—one step forward. I called my son, but there was no answer--two steps back. He called me. "Hey, Mama, how's your day?"—two steps forward—and I smiled. I called him, but there was no answer. I called him, and it went straight to voice mail. I called him; his phone was dead. Seven hours passed, and still there was no answer, still no response; four steps back.

Can your child possibly understand that you are in recovery along with them? Can they possibly understand or acknowledge that addiction is a family disease?

Our children's struggles become our struggles; their addiction becomes our addiction. Their addiction hurts their body; our addiction hurts our soul. Is their addiction different from our addiction? Of course it is. Do we fight, struggle, and suffer the pains of withdrawal? Yes, we do.

Is our withdrawal different from their withdrawal? Yes and no. They are in pain; they need counseling to understand their need for their substance of choice. They ache, they sweat, and they lie to cover up their addiction.

We are in pain; we need counseling to understand the need for their substance of choice. We ache, we sweat, and we lie to ourselves and withdraw from family and friends, in order to cover up that which we do not fully understand.

We too become addicts, not by choice but through determination to find resolve. We become addicted to meetings. We become addicted to finding answers—any answer that will help us to sleep through the night. We are addicted to the drive, to the devotion, and to the urgent need to solve this issue so we can go back to the life we once had. Though I don't believe we ever truly do.

Every day is a new day, and the sun does shine, but dark clouds loom closely in the background. Every time my child doesn't answer when I call, doesn't show up for work, or fails to arrive on time for a family event, I take a step back in my recovery. My addiction never ends; therefore, I turn to my higher power, and I seek answers from those who have traveled this path before me. We must support one another in our efforts to overcome that which addiction has caused.

Together, we can heal. Together, we can find our answers. Together, we will find new beginnings

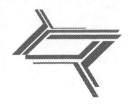

# Where Do We Turn

**W**here do we turn when the road ends? Where do we turn when it feels as though no one cares or understands? Where do we turn when friends turn their backs on us, and rehab is not working? If you have the answers, then you need to step up. If you have the ideas or solutions, then you need to share them.

The road from addiction to clean, for many, is difficult at best and downright impossible for some. Recovery and sustained sobriety is difficult, but it is possible. Still, the work it takes to get there will be one of the most difficult jobs a parent will ever face.

Many believe that addiction is a chosen path—a weakness, a moral failing, or a party for anyone willing to enter. If you believe this, then you have never been on the receiving end of addiction, especially in your child. Any parent with an addicted child will tell you that it is a nightmare that never ends. Even if your child is lucky enough to find his way back to clean, the fear of loss never ends for you, as a parent. You wonder if addiction will return or if your child will be gone tomorrow. God help me; I cannot breathe.

We need to offer more advice, and we need to find better ways to help parents dealing with addiction in their families. The number of children we've lost since September 2012 (when I began writing my journal) is far too many, and far too many more, sadly, will follow.

When parents are shaken to their very core, they seek help from anyone willing to listen. But far too many parents are left with feelings of isolation when their calls are not returned. What happens to families when they can't afford treatment for their children? What happens to families when legal counsel is not available and their children are facing criminal charges associated with the disease of addiction? Sadly, these two situations often go hand in hand.

I don't have the answers—maybe no one does—but I have to believe there is a way to provide better support and better assistance than what currently is in place. I have to believe there is a way to reach every parent who needs help, before it's too late to offer help. And I have to believe that every child in jeopardy of losing his battle with addiction must be offered a way back—before he finds a fatal way out.

If you know of someone who needs help or information, please do not ignore it. The response you offer just might save the life of an innocent child.

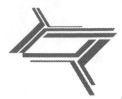

# UNTIL WE MEET AGAIN

I have been writing stories and letters and posting articles on the subject of addiction for nearly three years. I have learned about addiction and teen problems and almost too much about the pressures and coping skills needed when dealing with the disease of addiction.

Last week, I met a woman while I was shopping at the local grocery store. The woman intrigued me, because she smiled every time she placed items such as cookies, ice cream, and other wonderful treats into her cart. I have a very inquisitive nature, so I simply had to ask, "Why do you smile at the food you place in your basket? Can I ask the story behind your smile?"

I was unprepared for the exchange of dialogue that followed. As we left the grocery store, she said, "I will tell you my story." She then asked me to follow her to her home, and so I did.

She invited me in for a cup of tea. After she served the hot tea, she pulled out a video and said, "Let me show you something." The video was a slide show of her son, Jeffrey. The first several slides depicted an adorable and very cute baby. The women narrated, "Here is my Jeffrey at three months of age. He had just learned to smile." The next slides showed Jeffrey at one year of age; he had just learned to walk. This was followed by another sweet picture of Jeffrey at five years of age; he was playing piano—and playing brilliantly.

The women smiled and continued with her story. "Here is Jeffrey in high school—the star football player, the homecoming king, and the valedictorian of his senior class." Jeffrey had been accepted to an Ivy League college, where he'd planned to study medicine.

"After high school graduation," she then said, "Jeffrey attended a party. He came home drunk. I was surprised by his actions, because Jeffrey always thought it was dumb to drink, especially to drink enough to get drunk. But the next day, after a long talk, Jeffrey said, 'Don't worry, Mom. All the kids do it, and I have college plans, so don't worry about me.' That was in June 2007."

"By Fourth of July weekend, Jeffrey had attended nearly twenty more parties, and he drank at nearly every party. Then one night, Jeffrey came in, but he was not drunk—he was high, and all I could do was cry. The next day, Jeffrey said, 'Don't worry, Mom. All the kids do it, and I have college plans, so don't worry about me.' I grilled my son over and over. Concerned, I told him I thought he needed help. He became angry and said things to me that he had never said before. He took off, slamming the door behind him.

"On August 17th, just seventy-two days after Jeffrey graduated high school, Jeffrey, my sweet, beautiful boy, overdosed and died."

Jeffrey had left his mother a note, which she shared with me. She asked that I post the note on a message board or publish Jeffrey's words, with the hope that it might help someone.

> My dear mom,
> Oh, how you must be so disappointed in me. I have failed your expectations for my future. I have failed my own expectations as your son. I had fun at the parties this summer, and I believed I was not in any trouble; my drinking was just for fun. But Mom, one night a friend of mine (who, in reality, was not the friend I thought he was) introduced me to heroin. I thought to myself, *Yikes, no thanks, buddy. I pass.*
>     But then we smoked it, and I felt great! Later that night, I thought, *Okay, not too bad.* That was in June. Mom, by July 4th

weekend, I needed a fix so badly that I found my way to using a needle. I cried as I injected the heroin, but I was too afraid to say, "Mom, I need help."

Now, it is August 17ᵗʰ, I am starting college next week, and I know there is no way I will ever make it. I love you, Mom, and you need to understand one thing: this is all on me, and you did everything right. Please don't blame yourself for any of this.

I will always be with you, Mom, and when you go to the grocery store, you will see my smiling face in all my favorite foods, like ice cream and cookies. One day, Mom, we will share them again in heaven.

Until we meet again,
Your loving son, Jeffrey

I was in tears as she finished her story. Finally, I asked her, "How do you go on? How do you smile at the thought of simple food items in the store?"

She smiled back and said, "My Jeffrey was a beautiful boy, but he made some poor choices. I believe he would have been a great doctor, and he would have helped many people. I miss him every single day that he is gone, but my love is so strong that he is never too far away from my heart."

As I was leaving her house, we hugged, and she told me, "Please share my story as often as you'd like. Other parents need to understand that drugs have no boundaries. They require no prerequisites, and they will take anyone—their door is always open."

Many parents believe that only "bad" kids; wild kids or unsupervised kids get into drugs. Many children are too ashamed to seek help and too afraid to tell their parents that they need help.

Learn to recognize the signs of drug abuse, and then tell someone that you need help for your child. Don't let fear stop you from seeking treatment. And don't be afraid to say, "My child is in trouble. Can someone please help me?"

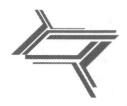

# IF I ONLY COULD

I f I could change the world, what would I change? How would I make the world a better place to live? What would I do that would change where I am today?

I have been a mother for more than thirty-eight years, and I am still perplexed when approached with questions of how I might change the world. You have to start small, with the things in your life that you can actually control or change. For me, life is measured one day at a time, one hour at a time, or perhaps one moment at a time.

My beautiful, brilliant son, who is now a young man, made some poor choices in his life as he ventured into the world of adulthood. I like to think that I could have stopped him from making those poor choices, but the reality is that I probably could not have done so. Today, my son is paying a very high price for his poor choices, and there is nothing I can do—except continue to love and support him. We can only control ourselves—and, at best, the moment or space we currently occupy.

Nine hundred sixty-three days ago, my life changed. Nine hundred sixty-three days ago, I learned that my son had an addiction problem, and nine hundred sixty-three days ago, my path in life was forever altered. My life, which seemed carefree, stress-free and normal by comparison, was altered by a world I barely knew existed. And it quickly spiraled out of my control.

As parents, we cannot prevent what we cannot see coming. Most of us did not recognize the signs of addiction. Many believe addiction is a choice, an open invitation to be accepted or declined. It is not. Addiction is a disease, however, not a choice. Addiction is a road without warning signs. I don't believe that anyone looks addiction in the face and says, "Wow, sounds like fun. Count me in." They have no idea of the journey the disease of addiction has in store for them.

If you change one thing about your past, would it change the things you cherish most? Life is a guessing game. You can change your current path, but you cannot change that which you do not see coming.

Albert Einstein once said, "The definition of insanity is doing the same thing over and over and expecting different results." Ask yourself, "Does this apply to the way I am living my life?" Have you been doing the same thing over and over and expecting different results?

I have watched as my son struggled toward the road to recovery, knowing full well that this road is never ending. Addiction will always have a place in my life, and it will always have a place in my son's life. Addiction is part of the past, but addiction always will be part of the future. I cannot control my son's addiction just because I am aware of what addiction is capable of doing. But I can offer him treatment and give him continued support on this long road ahead.

Keep in mind the simple rule of the three C's. The value of the most important letter in the alphabet (when addiction is on the table). I did not *cause* it; I cannot *control* it; I cannot *cure* it. Take care of yourself. If your child is suffering the ill effects of addiction, then treatment is usually the first line of defense. The effects of addiction, however, have altered your life as well, and you need to find your own form of treatment. Never allow anyone to devalue your needs. Support groups offer parents a place to vent, to rest, and to seek comfort in the knowledge that you are doing everything you can for your child. Now, however, you must seek comfort for your needs.

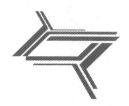

# In My Mind, I'm
# Already Packing

When we want to make a change in our career, we might buy a new outfit. We often jump in with both feet and eagerly seek a way to get what we need in order to make this change. We plan and schedule in our needs. We factor in the odds and open our minds to the possibility of success. Some changes can be achieved in minutes, and some changes require careful planning.

Addiction requires a lifestyle change, and it requires more planning than most people can begin to envision. Addiction requires factoring in the odds for success and the ability to open one's mind and think "outside the box."

Since February 2010, I have had a lifestyle for which I was unprepared, where tomorrow counts more than a million yesterdays. I surrounded myself with the possibility of loss of life, and I have learned of personality changes that have forever altered my existence. I learned of my child's disease of addiction, and I learned that the life I once had is gone forever.

While much of what I write these days are stories filled with the hope for a better tomorrow, I also write with great passion about the needs and support of parents—the need to mentor ourselves and the need to seek our own support system. If someone you love is seeking support or treatment, let him or her know that the Internet is filled with great information. Many parents, however, overlook the need for support for themselves. I was one such parent. Not too long ago, I believed there was no way to end my fear or anxiety about my child's disease. I was certain there was no way my life would ever go back to "normal." And there was no way I could face tomorrow, knowing my child might lose the battle before his recovery set in.

There is no way for parents to look forward without looking back. There is no way that parents can prepare for loss of their child's life. But there are ways to find resolve. It takes time to find your way back to normal. It takes time to find the peace of mind you once had. In my mind, I'm already packing. I am making plans for a brighter tomorrow, and I am making plans to seek a lifestyle change for me as well as for my child. You have to open your mind to the possibility of a brighter tomorrow.

Children learn much of their behavioral patterns from their parents and personal environment. They watch their parents' every move, and they learn from what see and hear. Their addiction has changed our road but hopefully not our path. I don't know if my fear of loss will ever leave my side, but I am eager to seek a healthier road for myself, with the hope that my child will follow in my footsteps. I am willing to seek support for my needs and not feel selfish in my determination to find a place to rest my thoughts.

When faced with any new challenge, we must be willing to face the idea of change. Change can only occur when we open our minds and realize that our children's addiction has forced us to face that which we never considered—the possibility of life without them.

My challenge for you today is simple: make a plan, find a way to put your plan into action, and then seek guidance for your own resolve. Are you up to the challenge?

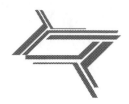

# A Day of Thanks

T oday is Thanksgiving Day. I am happy that my family is safe. I am thankful that my son is clean and sober, and I am glad that many of my family members and friends are supportive.

It would be a wonderful world if all of the above statements were true. Sadly, many are not. Yes, my child is safe, and yes, he is clean and sober—today. I am happy that the rest of my family is safe today, but tomorrow is not promised to anyone. No matter your faith, no matter your bank account, and no matter your race, tomorrow is a gift yet to be unwrapped.

I am truly sorry for the many families dealing with the fallout associated with the disease of addiction. I have been there, and in many ways, I will always be there. I recently met with a mom who had the courage to reach out; she is the mother of a teenage addict, and many family members have turned their backs on her. An aunt has turned away, because her son "might be a bad influence on his cousins." An uncle sees her son as a threat to his own children: "What if he turns them into addicts too?"

This mother was alone during the holiday season—without a sister, brother, or parents to help her to heal—because the family told her, "Leave the boy at home and join our family holiday dinner without him. He is not allowed in our homes. He needs to feel the consequences of his actions."

Can you imagine the pain, isolation, and hurt of such ignorant behavior from one's own family? Oh, how addiction destroys all in its path. It comes at a very high price—the loss of your family and valued friendships.

It does not make it easier to acknowledge that other families are facing the same hurtful behavior. It makes it more painful, as family should be there for each other, especially in a time of need.

How can you forgive your family when your child is considered to be the problem? I choose to believe it is *not* a problem; addiction is classified as a disease—a disease that is *not* contagious. Addiction is a disease that has entered the body of your beautiful child, and it destroys more than just its intended victim, a child caught off guard. The disease of addiction destroys entire families.

I wish I could wrap my arms around every child who is consumed by the disease of addiction. I wish I could share a meal with every child who has struggled to overcome the disease of addiction. But I cannot wrap my arms around the many who suffer from the disease of addiction, because the numbers are growing faster than my arms can reach.

My hope is that family and friends find the strength to not pass judgment. My hope is for the wisdom to help a lonely child to understand why his family has turned away from him. My hope is that one day we may welcome back those who turned away from us in our time of greatest need.

I hope you find the strength to see beyond the ignorance of family and friends. If your child is still with you, I hope you find the strength to hug your child. Tomorrow holds the unspoken promise of a better future.

We need to educate those who consider addiction a weakness and who see an addicted young soul and walk the other way, without offering support. We need to educate those who fail to understand that addiction is a disease and that there is hope of recovery. That recovery—known as remission—requires the love and support of family and friends in order to keep the disease in a state of remission.

Stay clean, stay safe, and stay sober. Post your needs on a message board; someone will hear you. Remember, for all those who turned their backs and walked away, there are others who are eager to stand by your side. Never give up hope!

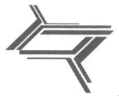

# IF YOU DON'T LIKE THE
# SCENERY, TRY CHANGING LANES

C hanging lanes is an experience in and of its self. Last week I changed lanes. However, I did not foresee the new scenery and I found myself unintentionally lost!

Like many people, I drive home from work following the same basic route on most days. I drive in the second lane of a four-lane highway, merely out of habit. I also focus most of my attention on what is right in front of me, with the exception of an occasional glance to my right.

Last week, however, while traveling the same highway I take nearly every day, I had the pleasure of my son's company. "Hey, Mom, move into the carpool lane; it's faster," he said, and so I did. I continued to focus my attention on what was in front of me, with the occasional glance out my side window. But this time, my glance was focused to the left—maybe it was the closest view and the glance was unintentional, but the scenery took me by surprise. I said to my son, "Where the heck are we?"

In a panic, I quickly looked to the upcoming street signs and realized I was still heading in the right direction, but I could not get that strange vision out of my mind. The scenery seemed unfamiliar to me. Why had I never noticed the left side of the highway? Are we really such creatures of habit that we fail to notice the unfamiliar? I guess I am.

As we continued our drive home, I found myself wanting to know more about the "left side of the highway." Were there more things I had overlooked in my life? Was I missing something important in my life?

I spent the next few days trying to uncover the mystery, the missing scenery of my life. I needed to make sense of this new concept and find out if there was more to this theory—and if I was the only person considering such a notion.

I suppose we could drive ourselves crazy, trying to explore everything we may have missed in life, simply because we were creatures of habit or had a fear of the unknown. Was I living my life out of choice, or had I become a creature of my habits? Do we form habits that keep us from a fuller life?

Some habits are fine and offer a sense of stability, but other habits can destroy our lives. Addiction is a habit without a reward. Addiction offers narrow roads, narrow focus, and limited options. My son's addiction came out of nowhere, and it took him on a journey without a reward. What started as a way to escape his demons quickly turned into a nightmare known as, addiction.

Today, I ventured out of my comfort zone. Today, I looked to the left, and I found a wonderful recovery treatment center for my son. Your recovery plan is out there, too, but you may need to change lanes in order to find it.

If you find yourself questioning your routine, habits, or predictable lifestyle, perhaps it is time to change lanes—to look in the opposite direction for your answers. Perhaps it is time to change your habits, before they become a way of life. Just a thought!

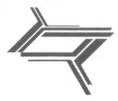

# COUNTING BACKWARD

When life throws you a curve, you may count the days until normal sets in again. When a child is born, we count their age in months until twenty-four, and then we count their age in years.

At age two, he took his first steps. At age three, he learned to run. At six, he joined karate, and at nine, he made first-degree black belt. At sixteen, he realized his first true love, and at nineteen, he realized his first broken heart.

Counting in days, weeks, months and years, the time slips away, yet we continue to count as though time will never run out. Time does run out for many parents who are dealing with the disease of addiction in their child or other loved one. I count the days that have passed since I first learned of my son's addiction (1,067 and counting). Today, however, the counting has changed for me—I count the number of days my son is clean.

I wake up, and I count the days since my life changed and my son began his battle to stay clean. I count backward on some days (the days my hands tremble, and the fear of loss consumes my very soul). However, I count forward to an event planned in the near future, and I smile with the hope of seeing my son alive and well. It is a strange way to live, yet it is my life. Many who have not faced the disease of addiction in a loved one find it sad; I count backward, to the exact day when I learned of my son's addiction; his disease, though there are as many who understand my need to count backward, as they too are counting backward on tough days and forward on good days.

I wish I had a crystal ball, and I wish I could tell you that one day this nightmare will be over, that one day addiction will no longer consume our every thought or take the life of another child. But I cannot tell you this any more than I can stop counting. We are, however, making progress in our fight to end or prevent the disease of addiction. With each story we share, other parents will find their way back to normal—by way of our declaration to find resolve. We have more parents standing up against the disease of addiction today than ever before. By sharing our stories, we have the power to lessen the burden faced by someone who suffers the ill effects of the disease of addiction.

We need to continue to educate our children, our loved ones, and our friends and family about the disease of addiction. We need to stand by our friends in need of support, for their battle should never be fought in isolation or shame. We need to remember why we post on social media sites like Facebook to express our concerns about addiction—we do this so other parents may learn from what has helped us to move forward.

I look forward to the day when I can count only the positive days ahead of me. I look forward to a time when I've forgotten the number of days since I first learned of my son's addiction. I look forward to sharing my life with anyone in need of guidance ... and I look forward to hearing the good that has come from a parent whose child has come through the maze and the nightmare of addiction—the day that child found his way back to clean.

For me, for today, I still count backward, but tomorrow ... who knows?

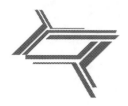

# I'll Take That
# Risk for You

*And the day came when the risk to remain tight in a bud*
*was more painful than the risk it took to blossom.*
—Anais Nin

This quote came to me today, and it made me realize that we are on the right path, perhaps for the first time in a very long time. We are going in the direction we were meant to go.

Addiction is like a bud, and many of us are too afraid to stare it down, too afraid to look it in the eye and say, "No more. No more will you take my child on a ride to nowhere. No more will you have access to my soul or try to lock me away and make me too afraid to speak about what you are capable of destroying. No more will you intimidate me into believing I am powerless in your realm. No more."

As we begin to fight back with a greater intensity than ever before, we begin to see the blossom of our strength. The pain has been hidden far too long; it is time to take back control. I have stated many times that we are greater in strength when we are greater in number. Now is the time to gather our strength. Now is the time to draw from one another's strength, as the strength in numbers is very powerful.

I have been terrified these past few months, as my son fell victim, once again, to relapse. I have felt defenseless in my ability to help him, as all I have done to date seems futile against such an enemy as addiction. I know the pain, the "bud"—afraid to share too much information with friends, as they may not understand my purpose. They may offer no more than a pathetic tilt of the head. Sometimes it is easier to "remain tight in a bud";

sometimes it is more painful to open up and risk the blossom, and so I shut down and isolate.

Can I hold true to my mission to end the war on drugs? Can I possibly gather enough willing soldiers to help me in this fight? I don't know. But we have lost far too many innocent children and young adults to this senseless, vindictive enemy. I do know that nothing will happen if no one steps up and willingly says, "I will risk the pain it will take to blossom."

I am willing to take a chance and to risk the pain of failure, as success is not measured in the number of failed attempts; success is measured in the number of willing souls it takes to fight back. I will take this risk for all parents who have lost a loved one to the disease of addiction. I will take this risk for my child and the many others who continue to fight for survival against the powerful force called, addiction.

Will you join me in this fight?

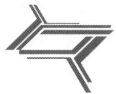

# THE VALUE OF A SIMPLE PIECE OF GUM

The value of chewing gum—what an interesting thought. How does one place value on chewing gum? I've never thought of a piece of chewing gum as anything of real value – poor thing, reduced to intangible item on the shelf.

Although, I would have to say the mere fact that I have chewing gum in my purse, in my car, and in my home at all times must mean something.

I chew gum for a particular reason these days. I chew gum to occupy my mind while watching my son struggle through the lessons brought forth from the disease of addiction.

My son suffers the disease of addiction; he suffers immensely from this debilitating disease. Sometimes he suffers alone in a dark corner, and other times he suffers while in treatment, yet somehow he's still alone. I chew gum to pass the time left at the end of my workday. I chew gum as a way to help alter the mood that accompanies my son's addiction. And I chew gum to keep myself from falling apart as my day slips into night, as I slip quietly into my dreams—though today my dreams have been altered as well.

At a recent support group meeting, I asked, "Anyone care for a piece of gum?" The room was filled with a show of hands, all requesting a simple piece of chewing gum. How strange that I would feel a welcome connection with my new friends via a piece of chewing gum. As we started to unwrap our pieces of gum, smiles came across the room. Maybe the flavor brought a pleasant memory of gum shared with a child, now gone too soon. But I also saw smiles from those who just enjoyed the uncomplicated pleasure of a simple piece of chewing gum.

Our world is forever altered when our children struggle with the disease of addiction. Day seems to melt into night before we even realize the day is over. Friends may try to offer support, but most cannot understand the complexity of addiction. Eventually, we drift off, and we are again left with the memories of a life now changed or a child gone too soon.

Thankfully, chewing gum is a staple that helps pass the time in this strange new world. Enjoy each moment that brings you a happy thought or pleasant memory. We deserve to find a moment of peace, no matter the instrument that brings us comfort—even if it's a simple piece of chewing gum.

Never underestimate the value of a piece of gum; a simple piece of chewing gum.

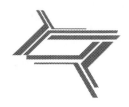

# I Had a Lovers'
# Quarrel Today

I had a lovers' quarrel with the world today, and I lost. I've played this emotion over and over in my mind, trying to retrace the steps I took that led me to where I am today. But I cannot find the footprints; I am stuck in today, and I want back my yesterday. I laid down the tracks of the type of life I wanted. I laid down the future I saw for my child. I made a plan and set this plan in motion—and now I can't stop the train with a one-way ticket to nowhere.

Addiction was not part of my plan, yet here it is. Addiction bought a ticket when I wasn't looking. Why didn't I see this coming? Addiction was waiting for the perfect moment to sneak in and rob me. This unwelcome, uninvited guest took my child and left me on the sidelines, watching like a bystander in my own life.

I recently read of a mom who took her life after the disease of addiction took her child, and I thought, *How selfish! She had another child still in the picture.* I pondered the battle she must have faced, a battle she thought she could never win, and again I thought, *how selfish.* But now, sadly, I understand.

Addiction never looks back; it only looks forward to the victory it hopes to win. A battle of this nature seems vague to those who are in their own safety net, thinking, *it cannot touch us; we've built a barrier out of steel.* Yet here it comes, with rules we cannot understand. Addiction has more patience, more power, and more backup plans than anyone could ever dream possible. Addiction is not afraid to strike when your back is turned. As a matter of fact, addiction usual does strike when your back is turned.

I need to retrace my footsteps before they fade away, before I see a future without my child. I had a lovers' quarrel with the world today, and I lost.

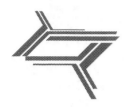

# Now You See Me

I see you; do you see me? Do you see me staring into your eyes? Do you see me watching you as though you might be gone tomorrow? Can I just hold you and pretend you're still my little child? Can I kiss your nose and still make you giggle?

When I saw my son the other day, I noticed that something in his face, in his eyes, was missing. What was it that I no longer saw? Why couldn't I see him looking back at me? Something was missing, and I want it back. I need to know that my child is still in there.

Addiction is a cruel and unforgiving disease, an illness that robs us of the child we gave birth to. Addiction was not invited, no matter what some may believe. My child would not have willingly entered this world; he was enticed by a power greater than his own, a power he never saw coming.

Someone recently said to me, "Why do kids do this to themselves? Why would they take such a chance with their lives?" My reply: "They didn't do this to themselves, at least not willingly." They did not foresee the end result. This was not what they expected. Would anyone honestly see addiction heading his way—see the pain and understand the consequences—and willingly open his arms to invite in such an evil monster?

I see what addiction has done to my child, and I want to scream. I want a way to fight back;. I want my child back, and I want addiction to pay the price for what it has taken from me and my child. But like many other parents, all I can do is pray that addiction doesn't come back and finish the job it so eagerly started.

Can you see me, baby boy? Can you find the strength to fight harder than you've ever fought before? Can I help you, my child? Can I lead you down a different path, and can I fight this fight for you? No, I cannot. I cannot do much more than what I'm already doing. This fight is your fight, so please fight, my sweet child, fight. Please come back to me!

I want to see your smile; I want to hear your laughter, and I want you to see me when I look at you. It is all I will ask of you. I want to count backward 1,565 days. I want to take your hand like I did when you were just a child, when I could say to you, "No, baby, not that way. Let's go this way."

I want … I need … I beg you … just come back.

I see you, my sweet child. Do you see me?

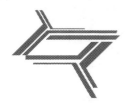

# YOU ARE NO MATCH

Addiction may be a bully, but we will not give up without a fight. So watch out, addiction, 'cause you ain't seen anything until you've seen us in action. Who are we? We are the parents of the children you've enticed into your club.

What can we do? We can do whatever it takes to run you out of our community. We won't play fair; we will destroy you and will leave a trail of destruction. Just like your own tactics, addiction, you will not see us coming. If you doubt our ability to take you down, then you have never seen a human chain—parents locking arms, with a grip so tight that nothing can penetrate our chain.

You've messed with our children for far too long; you've taken our young, innocent, and trusting children. But we no longer will sit and watch from the sidelines. We will invade your turf. We will intrude on your mission. We will be everywhere you are, and we have the will to protect our children at all costs. We will use everything in our power to break your hold.

We probably cannot save everyone currently caught in your grip, but we will win. We will take you down, and we will expose you for the fraud you are. We have a growing army of soldiers eager to fight this battle. We are our own weapons of mass destruction—we are parents, and you cannot compete with our force.

We will expose your dirty little secret, the line you feed to our children: "Come my way. I will show you to my party. Come with me on the ride of your life. You cannot escape. No one will love you the way I do." Lies, all lies—and we are on to you, addiction. And we have the truth on our side.

We will break your bond or die trying. We are taking back the power, even if that means sitting in a classroom and watching your every move. Even if that means sticking like glue to our children's sides. Even if that means standing next to our children to the point of being annoyingly embarrassing. We will do this, because we have that right, and we will exercise that right. We will take that chance because we are not afraid of you. We will not tolerate one more loss because of you. So watch out, addiction—your worst fear is about to become a reality. You have just met your match. We are called the PARENTS—

**P**articipant
**A**ggressor
**R**elentless
**E**ternal
**N**urturer
**T**imeless
**S**ustainable

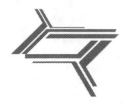

# WHERE IS MY RSVP

I received your RSVP, my child. You said, "Mom, I am on my way home. I will not disappoint you, Mama, not this time."

I received your RSVP, my child, and you told me, "Don't worry, Mama. I got this covered, and I know what I need to do this time." Your RSVP was in response to my invitation to regain your life.

It has been years, but not so many that the memories of yesterday have had time to fade. Do memories of addiction ever fade? I don't think they do. The painful memories do not fade for the addict, and they do not fade for the parents, as we push through the baggage left behind. A trail of victims follows addiction—casualties that latch on to everyone involved, and they latch on to some who were never part of the initial journey. Nothing good comes from the disease of addiction. Nothing!

I promised you, my child, a safe journey when first I met you, but now my invitation is once again sitting on a shelf, awaiting your RSVP.

Can you do it this time? Can you stay clean this time? Can I get through it this time? You have no definitive answers, nor do I. But we will try, one day at a time, one moment at a time, one prayer and one vow at a time. You will do your best, because you want a better life and a better future. I will ride this train with you again, because I promised you a safe journey, my sweet boy.

They call addiction a disease and indeed, it is. As with any disease, your life will forever be "one day at a time." And so, my sweet boy, together we will wait. We trust in God and we say, "We are stronger today than we were during your last remission." Maybe this time your disease will not win the war. Maybe this time we both will understand the rules of engagement when it comes to addiction. Maybe this time "our" addiction will take a backseat to the life we both want, the life we both deserve. Maybe. But for now, all I can do is sit here and await your RSVP.

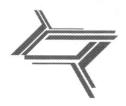

# I Am Paralyzed

I sit in my car, contemplating my next move, and I am paralyzed by what the disease of addiction has done to my life. Why me, why him, why any of us? There are no conclusive answers as to why this generation, more than generations past, has turned to drugs as a way to escape. Are they escaping that which life has failed to offer? I need an answer; we all need an answer.

Far too many have gone too soon, and others appear eager to line up and follow the same path. When a child or young adult says, with great passion in his or her voice, "I was not meant for this world," what can you do? Why do so many of our children seem so lost? What is happening to our youth today?

I search, I pray, I read, and I attend every meeting, every conference, and every workshop I can find, yet I sit in my car, contemplating my next move. I sit in my car, contemplating my child's next move, and I can no longer see my tomorrow—or his. I can no longer find the line in the sand, and so I cross over to the dark side to visit the world in which my child lives. It frightens me, and I beg for a way out.

So sad, some have said, that so many parents are contemplating their next move. So sad that we live daily with the fear of our children's next move, and yet we do. We have no choice, as we are now living with what addiction has done to our families, to our friends, and to our communities. Some talk about the "War on Drugs," but if addiction is considered a war, then where are the mighty troops to help us fight? Where are the financial resources needed to help us win this war? All I see are the casualties. All I feel is the pain. I do not see the end.

The cost to prosecute someone suffering the disease of addiction is higher than the cost of treatment. The cost to incarcerate someone suffering the disease of addiction is higher than the cost to rehabilitate. Hundreds upon thousands understand this, yet no one stepped up to change the system in time to save our children.

We edge closer to a solution with each new assembly bill, yet we still move too slowly to help those in desperate need. The current system is failing our children faster than we can save them. The current system is broken, and the bandage can no longer hide the open wound. The price of this war is the death of innocent, beautiful, and intelligent children—our children.

And so today, without a clear decisive plan, I sit in my car and contemplate my next move.

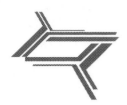

# A LIFE SENTENCE

The only life sentence I'm interested in is a life of prayer to end addiction. I cannot begin to imagine the pain of loss, because even though I have bad days, my son is still with me (today). The life sentence for those who have lost a child to addiction is a lifetime of tomorrows filled only with memories of a child gone too soon. Nothing is fair or just in that life sentence.

My heart feels your pain, and because of your pain, I can look in your eyes and tell you that I am fighting in memory of your loss. I am fighting to help my child find his way to clean. I am fighting this battle with the hope that one day soon, we will find a way to end this life sentence for other parents.

We fight together … until we win.

I am fighting this battle for those whose child is incarcerated and for those who are facing the idea of incarceration for the crimes committed because of addiction.

We are fighting this battle together, for the injustice of a jail sentence given for a disease that never should have invaded your child's life.

A life sentence? Yes, addiction is a life sentence, but it is one worth fighting against. We will not stop until addiction is far out of the reach of our precious children.

Give addiction the only life sentence it deserves, an unmarked grave where no child or parent ever visits.

# I Am Out of Words

I often write about hope for better days to come, but sometimes, there are no words left to write. There are no emotions, and there are no more dreams, for they too are gone. How can I keep going when my child's life never changes for the better? Addiction—I hate that word.

I once thought it addiction had caused my child's life to change. I once thought, *it's the disease that has robbed my child of his will to live.* But I was wrong. It was the drugs that caused him to live one more day. It was the drugs that took his pain away. How strange to even consider such a thought—but it is true.

How can I dream of a better tomorrow when my child's life is so gray or is it black? Does the color really matter? There is no drug that can truly hide his pain. Today he called and cried on the phone as he said, "Why, Mama, why did God make me this way?" He cried as he whispered the words, "I wish I had a way out of this life without hurting you. Oh, Mama, would you forgive me, if I were no I were no longer here? Please, Mama, just tell me I can go. Please tell me it's okay, and you will still love me. Please, Mama."

How can I survive the life that has come our way? How is this life fair, and why has God given my child this life? I have no more answers—not for you, not for me, and not for my sweet baby boy. I have no answers.

There are ups and downs in life, but today, they are all the same, and they have blurred into a world I can no longer explain. Was it the drugs that took him away? I don't know anymore. His mask is slowing dissolving into a person I no longer know.

He is unable to hide his pain. He can no longer hang on, waiting for a dream that never seems to come. And tonight, before he hangs up the phone, he says one more time, "Mama, please let me go, and tell me it will be okay."

And all I could think to say was, "Oh, my sweet boy, if you go, I go." I told him this because I am out of words. I told him this because I fear he will hear my innermost thoughts: *If you must go, my sweet child, I cannot stop you, but I do hope you will stay and let me continue to help you*. I cannot give him that much power. And so as I hang up the phone, I cry.

Maybe tomorrow will bring a new answer. Maybe tomorrow will bring a better solution to help us end this war. But for today, I am out of words.

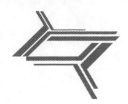

# If I Had a Dime

**W**hat truly defines us is how well we rise after we fall. What truly defines our character is our willingness to offer a second chance to someone who is facing the fallout that follows the disease of addiction.

Yet here I stand, catching teardrops in my hands, as I watch my son—and so many like him—be judged for a disease he could not control. Yes, he put the substance in his hand the first time, and yes, he took that unknown chance with his future. But he has paid a high price for his choices every day since then. So please, do not judge him.

Over the past four years, I have learned a great deal about the disease of addiction. As well, I have learned much about my son, myself, and those in my circle on whom I can count as true friends. I've heard more times than I care to admit, "Why don't you walk away? Get your life back, and go back to happier times."

Well, if life was just that easy, maybe I could go back to simpler times. Maybe I'd just wish away the past four years and start over, if I could. If any of us could, would we go back to life before addiction? Of course we would. I have yet to meet a single person who would answer that question with a resounding no. But life is not that easy, and sadly, we are judged for our choices and the choices of our children. We are only as good as our last time at bat—a baseball metaphor I have come to despise.

Children spend the first part of their young lives learning to be respectful of others. We teach our children the difference between right and wrong, and we teach them to forgive those who have made poor choices. As a mom, I have said more than once to my son, "I'm sorry; do you forgive Mommy?" And he always responded, "Of course I do, Mommy, I love you." I know I've heard my son say to me, "I'm so sorry, Mom; do you forgive me?" I have whispered in his ear many, many times, "Of course I do, baby; I love you." But what happens when life throws us a curve? What happens when our children realize that no matter how much they may have accomplished in their earlier years, they are only as good as their last time at bat. What a terrible quote to live by.

Of all the parents I have met whose children suffer with the disease of addiction, none has walked away. Not one has given up on their child out of the fear of what others might say—although I did overhear a parent ask, "How can you forgive him when he failed your expectations?" That question is wrong on so many levels. I cannot imagine my child failing my expectations, but what I can imagine is the pain *he* has endured, now that he has come in contact with the unfortunate and often deadly disease of addiction.

Yes, those of us living with this nightmare live it alongside of our children. We understand that addiction is a disease of the brain, a chemical imbalance. It's a disease so strong that it stands a great chance of winning the battle and taking our children from our arms. Still, we don't give up, and we don't walk away. We stay in the battle with them because they are our children.

If I had a dime for every time I heard someone say, "Just walk away," I would be rich. So today, I am still here, still fighting this battle beside my child. And at this moment, my child is still here, still alive—many parents cannot say the same.

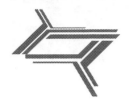

# I MISS THE SILENCE

Someone recently asked me what I missed most, now that my life has so drastically changed. I thought carefully on how to respond. And then I realized—I miss the silence at 3:00 p.m.

In my mind, I returned to 2004 or was it 2005, when my son was still in school—back to a life that seemed simple. I hadn't thought about those days as being simple by nature; they were just days on a calendar.

Now that addiction plays a significant role in the direction of my day, I've come to miss the moment of silence at 3:00 p.m., just before my son got home from school. Little did I realize at the time that waiting for my son to walk through the door would be something important enough to become a memory that I would one day beg to have back.

I miss idle conversations about homework, dinner menus, or clothes that needed to be washed—the blue shirt, because the girl he liked at school loved that blue shirt. ("Mama, I forgot to tell you that I need my blue shirt for tomorrow. Please, Mama, I will love you forever.") And so I did what many moms have done—I smiled and said, "Okay, I will wash your blue shirt"—even though it was nearly midnight. Oh God, how I miss the little things.

I miss writing my to-do list for the next day. I miss conversations on the phone with a friend in the evening, once my son was tucked safely into bed. Today, I hate the silence at the end of my day, and I hate that most of my friends have since left my side.

Today, my days are filled with anger, resentment, and guilt—guilt over what I might have failed to see coming. Today, my days are filled with; what-ifs and why-nots. And today, my days are filled with so much confusion. There are not enough hours in a day to finish even the first page of my to-do-list.

I am planning to move to a smaller home, and I have approximately thirty days to do so. I am moving because when my son gets out of jail, he and his girlfriend want to start their new life together in my home. I cannot say no to him, because this is the one dream to which he is clinging. Moving into my home is the only plan that is keeping him focused.

I can't remember the last time I moved just for me. I have no idea how to do something just for me without feeling guilty. Addiction is the newest member of my household, and I am trying to find a way to ask it to leave. I need addiction to forget my address, forget my phone number, forget my name, and forget my child's name. I need addiction to move out of my home as quickly as it entered.

I miss the good silence, and I hate the sad silence. I hate my idle time, and I want back what I once thought of as a normal life. Even if I become one of the lucky parents whose child makes it through the dark door of addiction, addiction will always be lurking in the background, eagerly waiting for the perfect moment to sneak back into our lives.

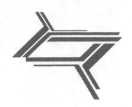

# A Battle without an End

Every battle has casualties. Some casualties are visible, and some are not, but all are casualties of the heart. Addiction is a war without an end in clear sight. Although addiction is fought all over the world, when the battle of addiction is fought in your home, the fight to win becomes personal.

Some wars are fought with one purpose in mind, while other battles exist only to prey on the weak. Our children are fighting a war in which the enemy is nearly invisible—until it grabs their souls and refuses to let go.

Many people believe addiction has willing participants—eager members looking for a thrill. Many believe the weak, the wild, or the rebellious child seeks out addiction. ("They got what they asked for.") Some have paid with their lives, while others appear to have survived, but they have paid with their souls and with their future existence.

We could turn a blind eye and say, "Not in my family. This doesn't affect me. My kids are smarter than that." But who are we trying to kid? In today's society, you'd have to be deaf and blind not to realize that addiction is a master manipulator with the patience of a saint. Addiction is willing and able to wait for the most curious and innocent minds. These underdeveloped, innocent, curious minds are now soldiers in a war without an end in sight.

If you think the phrase "the War on Drugs" is just a media statement to grab attention, then you have not been paying attention to the world around you. Addiction may be classified as an epidemic that is out of control, but it is an actual *war*—a world war—and there are many casualties. There is loss of life, and there are those left behind to grieve the loss of an innocent child. We need to fight hard to regain control. We cannot allow this war to continue to take our children. Addiction is a war without clearly defined rules. The disease of addiction has no honor, no badge of courage, and no medal for a job well done. There are no winners in the war of addiction, only victims. We cannot let this war become a fatal attraction for another innocent child or unsuspecting young adult.

Educate your children, but also educate yourself on drugs and addiction, so you have a defense plan prepared, should addiction try to enter your child's world.

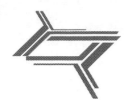

# TELL ME I'M WRONG

I wish I didn't know what drugs might one day take from me. I wish I didn't wake up in a panic from the nightmare that plays over and over in my sleep, where drugs already have taken my child. Tell me I am overreacting and that addiction has an end that leaves my child intact, as though addiction were just someone else's nightmare.

Even on my good days, my heart hurts. Even when my son calls and says, "Love you, Mom," my smile quickly turns to fear—what if that's the last time I hear him say those words? I know that the possibility of death rides too close to the surface. Others tell me to take it a day at a time. I miss the days when I thought addiction happened to others but not to my child. I miss the days when a nightmare could be dispelled by waking up.

Tell me I'm wrong to spend so many hours of my day in fear of what might happen. Tell me I'm wrong, and one day I will look back on this experience and not remember, in great detail, the relapse, the overdose, or the near-fatal moment in my son's life. Please tell me that the years ahead will outnumber the addictive years of the past.

Today was a good day—until I found out that a close friend to my son had relapsed. After nearly two years of sobriety, he now can no longer count the days ahead; he must count backward to square one. I have not told my son of this current event, as I fear it will hinder his sobriety. It may cause him to rethink his mortality and his ability to maintain "clean." He counted on the continued "clean" of his dear friend. And so I fear the unknown—once again.

Addiction is the devil in disguise. Addiction is often invisible to even the most brilliant of our children. Our children are intelligent, creative, and sensible, so how is it that our advice to steer clear of this devil does not affect their decision to experiment? Why is addiction so powerful?

My only suggestion is to keep a watchful eye. Learn more about addiction and about street drugs or prescription drugs. Learn about the perils of experimentation; learn more than your child knows, so you are the one to whom he will turn when the thought of experimenting tugs at him. Be that person with whom your child feels comfortable enough to ask, "Mom, is this drug really safe to try?"

Do not be afraid to show your child the reality of addiction. Education and awareness is our *only* weapon against the disease of addiction.

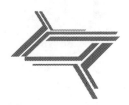

# I Saw Him Today

I saw him today—my son, my child. He is in jail, and as he sat on the other side of the table, he was disengaged in our conversation. Nothing can prepare us for that which addiction takes from us—it takes our children's souls.

Yesterday was a good day, and yesterday I loved the excitement in my son's voice when he called. I admired the enthusiasm in his plans for a better future, and I cherished his commitment to finding or re-finding that which now seems so far away yet again.

I knew his mood could change on a dime, just as it has done many times before; I was warned his mood could change on a dime just as it has done many times before. I knew better than to expect to see the smile on his face that I'd heard in his voice less than twenty-four hours earlier when we talked on the phone. I knew better, yet I hoped and prayed that I would see his eyes light up. But they did not. The look in his eyes scared me to death. It was a dark, disengaged look that said, *"Mom, things will never really change, will they?"* And so he fakes it. He pretends that I don't know what he's thinking, yet I do.

We hear the stories of "the look" from others who have been where we are now, yet we assume that our story will be different. We believe our child, now clean, has the whole world open to him, with opportunities waiting that will be enough to keep him on the straight and narrow … but it seldom is.

Addiction is a disease that takes the personality of our children and draws out every ounce of hope for normal. I know that many will make it back to "normal" with their brain cells intact, dreams intact, and have a future with a full view of possibilities. I also know that many do not make it back.

I saw him today, and now I have retreated back to my catacomb of panic. Addiction changed his life, but addiction changed my life as well. I am no longer the easygoing person I use to be. Addiction took away my ability to plan my future, since I cannot walk away from my child.

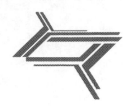

# It Happened on
# My Watch

I raised a sensible and intelligent child, a dreamer with a passion for life. He trusted that which he did not fully understand. I trained him—this little boy, this child with a dream—and I walked hand in hand with a child who was meant for so much more. Still, this happened on my watch.

What goes through the mind of an innocent child when a power greater than his says, *"Try me; trust me; I am exciting. I will give you wings. I can take you to a place where you can fly, and I will never leave your side."* Addiction has what most parents do not—a crystal ship with a vision of what you think you'll never achieve without the power of a substance. Addiction allows you to believe that you have choices, that you are in control, and that you can stop whenever you want. Addiction has an open-door policy, but often the door only swings one way.

As a parent of a child suffering the effects of addiction, you believe that you have the power to be more persuasive than the allure of the drug. Sadly, many times you are no match for addiction; your power is, at best, limited. You are only the parent; you had the power to heal the scraped knees and to wipe away tears when your child was sad. You had the power to heal the first broken heart when puppy love entered the game, but those powers are no match to the power of the crystal ship.

How could this choice take away the child who was yours only yesterday? How could the child you raised not understand that this new friend is anything but a friend? You never saw it coming; you never saw the outcome. How could this have happened on your watch?

How did this happen on my watch?

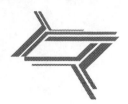

# I Believe In …

In 2010, I was shocked to learn of my son's disease of addiction and that his drug of choice was heroin. I believed that after treatment for ninety days, life would be back on track—train wreck diverted, home stretch just ahead. I was wrong on more levels than the princess who slept on the pea had layers of bedding. But still, I believed all things were possible.

I believe in happy endings. I believe in second chances, and third chances and fourth chances and fifth chances, and more chances than I can count. I believe in butterflies, and blue skies, and Boston cream pies. I believe that no soul is so far gone that a hug can't bring him back. I believe in a mother's touch and a stroke of luck, and I still believe in happily-ever-after fairy-tale endings.

I believe we can walk a mile in someone's shoes and still never understand that person's pain. Yet we try, because we need to see a black hole before we can surface to a new light. I believe there are people who come into our lives just to remind us to smile, no matter how sad we feel or how gray the future may look. I believe in hope, even when no one around me can see the light in my child's eyes. And I believe I will survive, no matter what tomorrow may bring, because I owe it to my child.

I believe that no matter the nightmare of yesterday's sorrow, I am here so I can hand someone else's child the hope of a better tomorrow. I believe addiction has an end, because I've already seen the beginning and the middle. I believe addiction is in our lives for reasons none of us will ever fully understand. And I believe that for many, the road back is possible, for reasons I cannot explain.

I believe I have seen the future. I have turned from the future, and I have walked back in time to see it happen again. I have seen the tears in a mother's eyes as she tries to hold tight to the memories of a child gone too soon. And I have felt the fear of my future, should my child's life follow suit.

I believe I will stay strong and count my blessings for a better tomorrow. I believe in water slides, and Moon Pies, and tears of joy and not good-byes. I believe there is a reason beyond what we can see. I believe in honey bees, and crisp white sleeves, and sandy feet, and an ocean breeze. And most of all, I believe that as difficult as life can be, the love we share with our children is still better than all the sad tomorrows.

And I believe the day will come when addiction is no more. I believe the War on Drugs will be replaced with a thousand hugs. I have to believe all of this, because the alternative is not working for me … and so for today, all I will say is,

I believe in …

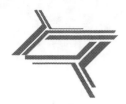

# THE DEMON WITHIN

The drug ... the choice ... the demon within. My child today is not the child I gave birth to. The choice that changed him snuck into his life, neatly wrapped and cleverly disguised—a disguise many intelligent souls have failed to recognize.

We teach our children many things as they grow into their own. We teach them to stay away from strangers—those disguised as nice people, such as the ice cream man, the postman, and sadly, even a police officer, because the boogieman has many disguises. The drugs that possess our children often sneak in through a friend, a "best" friend who smiled and said, "Here, try this. It will take your pain away. And by the way, don't worry. I do it all the time, and look at me. I am just fine." So they believe their trusted friend. That first choice is often their last *free* choice.

The drug is now the identity of your child. A few years back (and only a few months into this nightmare), my son ran away from his first treatment facility. He had relapsed; he had been given what is commonly known as a *hot shot* (a lethal amount of heroin), and he nearly died. When I found him and brought him back to the treatment facility, the director in charge asked him one question: "Why should I take you back?" My son broke down in tears, fell to his knees, and said, "'Cause I don't want to die."

After they took him back, I left him in their care and then drove to a quiet place, where I cried uncontrollably for nearly two hours. The child I left that day was not the child I gave birth to. My child was now the victim of the demon within. Three years later, he is still the victim of the demon. He is still the victim of one poor choice. Many unsuspecting parents assume this could never happen to their children. They assume their children are too bright to fall victim to the demon known as drugs; I know this to be so, because I too was once such a parent.

Three years ago, I said, "Not my child. He is bright, he is fun-loving, and he is grounded by the sports I enrolled him in. My child could never be fooled by such cleaver wrappings of the drug." God, how I wish that were so, yet here we are, battling this demon and all the baggage that follows. I still pray for a breakthrough that will save his life and return his soul. Is he clean today? Yes, he is. Is he free of his poor choices? No, he is not, and he may never truly be free from those choices.

Who do we blame when our children are lost? Can we blame the friend who initiated the path? Can we blame the doctor who offered medications never intended for a child? Can we blame the arresting officer who placed extensive and exaggerated charges on the victim, starting a new road to hell? Yes, we can blame them all, but unfortunately, it brings little comfort in return for what we've lost—our precious children. We've come so far, yet still we fail to understand the simple things.

We find little comfort or help when our children are caught in a cycle created by one poor choice. Addiction is a demon that fails to offer a way out, no matter how much we beg to be released from its hold.

When a community has more sober-living homes than grocery stores, we are in trouble. When every neighborhood has a treatment center, a detox house, a medical marijuana dispensary, or a probation office all within walking distance, we are in trouble.

I know this is wrong on so many levels. I am an advocate for better education and greater awareness to fight against drug addiction. But sadly, more teens and young adults continue to be fooled by this cleverly disguised demon.

Despite our best efforts, many continue to believe that drugs, when offered by a friend, are not dangerous. And so the battle begins.

Enter the demon within.

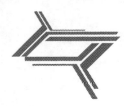

# You Have Three Minutes

I attended a meeting a while back and can only now put into words to what transpired that evening. This group meeting was dedicated to parents of children with addiction. I hoped I might learn something new that evening. And I attended because I thought there was nothing new I could learn about a parent's struggle with a child's addiction. I was right, and I was so very wrong.

The facilitator started the meeting: "Welcome, everyone, I hope tonight brings the message that addiction is a family disease, not an isolated affliction of your child." Everyone presented a typical introduction. "My name is … and my child suffers from the disease of addiction." Most everyone in attendance had similar stories. Tears fell; hearts pounded, and heads shook. Everyone asked the same questions: why my child? What could I have done differently? Were there signs I didn't see? Could I have stopped or prevented this terrible journey?

One parent told her story in a chronological fashion: "I was a mother at seventeen to a beautiful blue-eyed baby boy and on that day, my life began. Fifteen years later, almost to the day, my son turned to drugs. Life was on hold. But two years down the road, I got him back. Seventeen and seventeen—I was thirty-four with a seventeen-year-old son. Five years into sobriety, addiction caught him again, at a time of great weakness and vulnerability—a breakup with his girlfriend, the loss of his grandmother, and the loss of a dear friend to addiction. However, this time his addiction lasted twelve years, and today, he is once again clean. I am now fifty-one years old, and I still live in fear of where the next seventeen years will take us."

As the evening progressed, one woman sat silent each time the focus landed on her. The facilitator presented a new suggestion to the group: "I'd like to close with an unusual request." She took out an egg timer and said, "I'd like to go around the table and allow each person to say, in three minutes, what the disease of addiction has done to you, the parent."

Each person tried desperately to use every second of his or her three minutes; it was almost impossible to squeeze so much emotion into three little minutes. The last mom given a turn to speak was the mom who had said very little throughout the evening. Once again, the egg timer was set, and the attention centered on this mom. The room was silent; for three full minutes, the room was silent. She glared at the timer but never spoke a single word. The time ran out, the bell chimed and still, the room was silent.

Finally, she stood and spoke: "Addiction took the light from my son's eyes until there was no one on the other side looking back at me. Addiction took his smile until he could no longer smile. Addiction took his words until there were no words left for him to speak. And addiction took his heart until there was no sound left to hear, except the deafening sound of a flatline. So if I have three minutes to tell you what addiction has done to my life, there is nothing left of my child, except silence. So to answer the question, I guess I would have to say, addiction took everything."

She turned and left the room, and we sat in silence for what felt like an eternity. No one had a word left to add; she was right. Addiction robs us of the very things we love about our children, and addiction leaves far too much silence in our lives.

So now I ask you: if you had only three minutes to express what the disease of addiction has done to your life, what would you tell someone who was listening to—or clinging to—your words?

The timer is set; you have three minutes.

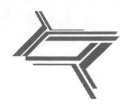

# THE BOY IN THE
# ORANGE JUMPSUIT

How often do we think about our future? How often do we visualize our future? As a young adult, did you imagine what your life might look like when you were grown and have children of your own?

Never in my wildest dreams did I consider the life my child would have if he did not stay on course with what society expected of him. Never did I envision my son in an orange jumpsuit. Never did I imagine speaking to him from behind a glass window on a telephone touched by thousands before me. Never, and yet the disease of addiction brought more what-ifs to my life than I could have ever imagined.

An orange jumpsuit was never part of my dream or any vision I had of my life or my child's life. Never … Never … Never …

Today, the boy in the orange jumpsuit is not my child, it is not your child, and it is not anyone's child. It is merely a consequence of a poor choice. It is the consequence of the disease, a disease that society fails to recognize, help, or acknowledge. The *American Journal of Medicine* tells me this is so, and yet society treats the person with the disease of addiction like a leper. "Send them off to a remote location, and let them die. Let them self-destruct." What a society we live in.

Perhaps part of the stigma stems from the term "addiction" or "addict" or "druggie." These terms depict a vision of a powerless, nonhuman soul, willing to steal, to cheat, to lie, or to kill for his next fix; the almighty high. But never, not once in my life, could I have imaged this road for my child. The orange jumpsuit is now the identity of far too many innocent lost souls. Where do we go for help when our beautiful, brilliant children are caught up in a system intended for those with no values? A place meant house criminals—thief, murderer, rapist, child molester. A place never intended for someone with a disease. A place where souls go to die and spirits are destroyed. A place with a revolving door—life on one side and hell on the other. Once they are caught in the system, few emerge cured of their disease. Sadly, many emerge more filled with the disease of addiction than when they entered. Drugs are available in jail. (Did you know that? I didn't.)

Our system is broken. Our system has failed our children. Our children have a disease; society calls it a disease. Yet society is willing to throw away our children like yesterday's rubbish. The disease of addiction has turned into a fight, a battle to find a better system—before there are no more tomorrows for our children.

Whatever you do, do not allow your child to become a victim "Of the Orange Jumpsuit."

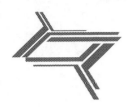

# Damn, I'm Out of Whipped Cream

Living life as the parent of an addict is more than any parent should have to bear. But sadly, we are many in number. You never know what the day will bring when the disease has your child. The uncertainty of the day can be the breaking point for many. Addiction is not for the faint of heart. Addiction is a disease, and yet the hope for a full recovery is a long, terrifying journey.

The day started like any other. I had the day off from work in order to get ready to move to a new apartment in a new area—a fresh start and a new beginning. When the phone rang that morning at 7:12, I saw my son's picture and his number flashing on my phone. My heart stopped, and I felt frozen in time. Only seconds had passed, yet it felt like a time continuum.

Although my son suffers from the disease of addiction, I suffer from the disease of fear, and the two go hand in hand. With only a few months of sobriety under his belt, when anything out of the ordinary happens, my first thoughts go to fear of relapse. As part of an early release from jail, my son is working off his remaining time in a community work program (CWP). He works Monday through Friday, from 6:00 a.m. to 2:30 p.m. He's not allowed to use a phone during work hours, so why was he calling me? *Dear Lord, just tell me what happened.*

As I reached for the phone, which now seemed to be ringing louder, I quickly said, "Oh God, baby boy, what did you do? What's wrong?" His voice was shaky, and as he started to speak, tears formed in my eyes, but

I still could not hear what he was trying to say. Finally, he said, "Mom, I don't feel well, and they are sending me home. Can you pick me up?"

It is now 7:20 a.m., only 8 minutes has passed since the phone rang, yet it feels like hours. As I hung up the phone, my knees started to buckle. The past four years of living in this nightmare told me that there might be more to this story. I quickly threw on some clothes, grabbed my keys, my phone, and my sunglasses—I needed to hide the fear in my eyes.

As I pulled onto the freeway, I noticed my blouse was on backward and inside out, and I was wearing two different shoes. I glanced in the mirror; I looked disheveled, like a homeless woman, but there was no time to turn back now. *"Watch the speed limit,"* says the voice in my head. *"Don't go too fast, but don't go too slow either."* Do I look suspicious? If I get pulled over do I confess; I'm on my way to get my son, and I think maybe he's high … or perhaps in trouble.

Finally, after what felt like hours but was, in reality, only thirty minutes, I pulled into the parking lot, where I saw my son waiting. He was standing in the cold, shivering, his hoody pulled over his head. He looked like he did in 2010 when I first learned of his disease. I pulled up, and he got in the car. He smiled and said, "Thanks, Mom, it's so nice and warm in here." Then he asked, "What's wrong, Mom? Are you sick too? You look a little pale." I stopped the car and said, "Look me in the eye. I need to see your eyes."

"I was sneezing and coughing," he said, "and they told me I needed to go home."

My hands stopped shaking. I looked at him and said, "Really, baby boy? You're okay? You're not high, and you're not in trouble?" He smiled again and replied, "Yes, Mom, I'm fine. I'm clean, and don't worry about me. I'm not in any trouble."

It was a good day. My Christmas wish had just been granted. Maybe this Christmas would be different. Maybe he would be clean this Christmas. Maybe he would be home this Christmas.

As we head toward his house he says, "damn, I'm out of whipped cream, can we stop and get some before you take me home, it sounds good right now." Whipped cream? Yes, my sweet boy, we can get some whipped cream.

Addiction … not for the faint of heart and never meant for our children, but now that addiction is here, it is always on the front burner. It is always where my mind goes first whenever my phone rings too early or too late in the evening. I have tried to keep addiction from destroying my life or my child's life, but that may take years to accomplish. On this day, however, I was willing to play along, because so far—for me, for my son—this was a *good* day.

As I walk back into my house, I reach for some Jell-O then I realize, "Damn, I'm out of whipped cream" … and I smile.

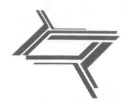

# TELL ME YOUR STORY

I met a person whose story validated my mission to write about my life, even when I don't want to write. It was a strange meeting, a meeting that seemed to be more of a destiny than a casual conversation between two strangers. The space in the heart of a stranger is almost more visible than that of a friend or a loved one in need.

The day was warm, though the clouds were dark and the wind was blowing. There was an empty seat on a park bench, where no wind or chill air could touch, and so I sat down. Seated on the other end of this bench was a stranger, a young man. Within minutes, I felt a sense of sadness float above this stranger, as though this sadness was meant to be visible.

I watched in silence, trying not to impose on the stranger's quiet time, yet I was somehow drawn to continue watching him. And so I continued to watch. I allowed this quiet time to settle upon the two of us like a protective shield, knowing we were meant to occupy this space together. After fifteen minutes or so into my meditative state, I heard the whisper of a small voice, and the silence was broken. I glanced to my right and met the eyes of the person whose heart shared this bench. I said, "I'm sorry. I didn't hear your words clearly. Were you were speaking to me?" His reply is where this story unfolds.

"Yes," said the stranger, "I was. I asked if you could you feel it too. Do you feel the emptiness, the void of the world? Do you feel it too?" I was taken aback by the question, yet not completely sure I was following him. Then I heard this soft-spoken stranger say, "I have seen more death than anyone should see. I have attended more funerals than a body should attend. And

I've hugged more people with broken hearts than I've hugged those whose hearts are happy."

The stranger's words continued to flow in a sad, almost poetic fashion. "I've bought more flowers for funerals than I have for weddings actually I've never been to a wedding. But I've heard they are fun." Then, suddenly, the conversation stopped. And once again, we sat in silence, and shared a bench in the park.

A few minutes passed before the stranger continued speaking. "I've dried more tears of pain than I have tears of joy. I've helped to pack up more personal belongings of someone gone too soon than of someone moving into a new home. I've served more meals to a family whose hearts were broken from pain than I have with families in need of a hot meal. And I have more friends gone because of a drug overdose than I have friends still standing near me. It would take more than two hands to count the number of friends who are gone too soon, but I need only one hand to count the friends who are still here."

I watched this stranger in silence, as I had no poetic words to share. And so we sat and enjoyed the warmth of the sun for several more minutes. We shared this bench, but I still was uncertain as to why this encounter had occurred. Was I meant to tell a story? Was I meant to share the words of this stranger with others?

It felt like hours had passed since our conversation ended, yet only minutes had surrounded us before I replied, "I knew you had experienced pain. I saw the pain in your eyes, though I was not sure what might have caused such pain. I too have seen this pain in others as I've watched and listened to countless stories in a special support group I attend. And I too have struggled with fear as I've watched my child struggle to find his place in this often chaotic world."

I continued my conversation with this stranger, who occupied the other end of the bench. "I write stories about the pain I see, the pain I feel, or the pain I witness in those around me. And sometimes, I want to run away and hide. I want to stop writing about pain and about fear. I want to write about happy times. I want to write about love or about a child's first steps. And sometimes, I want to stop writing altogether, but I can't, because there are so many stories yet to be told." At that moment, we both stopped talking and once again sat in silence, enjoying the warmth of the sun on a bench we shared in the park. I'm not sure why I shared this information with this young stranger, but I felt somehow compelled to volunteer my story.

It appeared we both had said what we needed to or were meant to say. At nearly the same moment, we stood up, looked into each other's sad eyes, and prepared to leave the park. As we stood in an almost awkward moment of silence, this stranger turned to me and said, "I am only sixteen years old, and this is not how my life was supposed to be. I don't think I am old enough to have witnessed so much pain in such a short period. I don't know what to do with what I have seen in this sad world." I turned and hugged this child. I felt the tears build up in my eyes, and I felt his pain in my heart. I now understood that the chance meeting with this young soul was not a chance meeting at all. It was a strange destiny for each of us.

As we parted, I offered these final words: "I know of some wonderful people who can help you to deal with or perhaps better understand what you've been through. I can give you some numbers." This young boy, only sixteen years of age, looked at me. He smiled a most beautiful smile, and he said, "That's okay. I just met one. I want you to write about me and my story, so maybe someone who reads the words will offer hope to a stranger in the park. I will be fine; I know there are better days ahead for me. I try to surround myself with positive people, but for many others, who have seen or witnessed this pain firsthand, there is only a dream of a better future."

I watched as this sixteen year old child walked away, and I cried. He was right. He was far too young to have seen or have witnessed so much pain. Still, he seemed to know there was the hope of a better life, especially if we show love and support to others in need and show that someone, even a stranger, cares about us. And so I will continue to write and share the stories of those I meet along the way as I journey through the world of addiction.

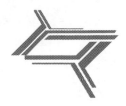

# I SAW A MAN TODAY

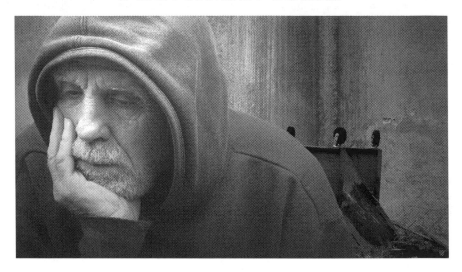

I saw a man today. He was cold and looked hungry and defeated by the world. He was sitting on the steps of the bank as I entered to make my deposit. He was still there as I came out of the bank, and he looked up at me and said, "Hi, how are you today?"

"I'm good," I replied. "How are you?"

"I'm good," he answered, "a little cold but good." Then he said, "You are the first person today that's asked how I am. As a matter of fact, I think maybe you're the first person in a very long time who has talked to me at all."

As I got in my car, I looked over at him again, but he had already lowered his head down into his lap. I rolled down my window and held out a twenty-dollar bill, saying, "Sir, please take this and buy a hot meal." He raised his head, stood up, and walked toward my car to accept the bill, but what happened next took my breath away.

As the man stood near my car, tired and disheveled, he glanced down at the bill I'd offered him and started to cry. I heard him whisper, "I can't take this much money."

"Yes, sir, you can," I insisted. "I want you to get something hot to eat and a hot drink."

He looked at me, and as he took the bill, he said, "I have never been called 'sir' in my entire life. I'm not sure I deserve such a title."

All I could say was, "Yes, you do. Everyone deserves respect." As I pulled away, the man stood tall, and he waved at me like a child would wave, with pure excitement in his movement.

I have no idea how the world got him to where he was that day. I've asked myself why we are here, and why so many are in such great pain. Sadly, I have no answers. I've begun to realize that we are surrounded by pain and misfortune. I'm not sure I enjoy being part of such a world. Perhaps the depth of my child's world is becoming my world.

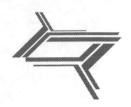

# WHERE IS MY ANGEL?

He was. He is. I am. We are. Words—just empty sounds that roll off my tongue, and I can't get them back, and he cannot say them, not today. He is not here, and I am not there, and I cannot remember when everything changed or how it changed. It seems like yesterday, yet it feels like a thousand yesterdays ago.

The questions I hear most often are, "How did this happen? Why did this happen?" I want my angel back—back the way he used to be. Is he gone forever, or just for today? Will he ever be back—all the way back? Will he stay this time, or will I lose him again? Empty thoughts filled with anger; it didn't have to be this way. We could have stopped it; they could have stopped it. But they didn't care, it wasn't their loved one, caught in a nightmare. They are the ones with the power to make a difference, and they didn't care. Politicians, legislators, doctors—those with the means and the power to influence society.

I heard of the loss of another sweet angel today. A life once filled with promise, gone too soon, and they could have stopped it. Was his name not big enough? Was he the product of ordinary people? Was his life not worth saving? How many have died, this early into the New Year? I think I counted twenty-five. We are only fifty days into the New Year, and already twenty-five are gone. We are losing one angel every other day. By the end of the year, we stand to lose 185 precious angels, but reality and history tell me that it will probably be many more. Will my child be one of them? Do they care?

We are losing an entire generation of brilliant, loving, sensitive angels; we are losing them. Our voices need to be louder, but still, only a few will be heard or acknowledged. We have ordinary last names, so we are disposable. They are disposable.

Where is my angel? Will he come back? I heard him cry out today, "*Mom, please save me! I can't do this again,*" and all I could say was, "I know, baby, I know. I love you." I can't save him; they can, but will they? Perhaps they would care if the disease of addiction took one of their angels, an angel with a name perhaps less ordinary. But for today, we wait, we cry … and I ask, "Where is my angel?"

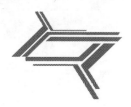

# KNOCK KNOCK

I woke up this morning, and before I opened my eyes, my mind whispered, *knock knock*—but no one answered. What a sad and strange way to begin my Monday. This was the thought in my mind that followed my opening dialogue with the day. How sad that the words *knock knock* came to mind. And sadder still, the idea that no one answered.

*Knock knock.* Who's there? Nobody. Nobody who? Hello, are you still there?

It was a weekend filled with fear, with tears, with regrets, and most of all, a weekend filled with, "Where in the world did my son go?" He is still here, at least in the physical sense. Sometimes, throughout the weekend, he was here both physically and mentally, but the changes in him these past few months are extensive. The darkness in his eyes, even when he's laughing, no longer scares me; it simply makes my heart stop beating. That distant darkness is enough to end my hope of a great future, for either of us.

Did the addiction do this to him? To me? Did the disease of addiction take the light from his eyes? Did the addiction take me to a place I now call home? Yes, and no. As my son as has told me many times in the past, "It was never about the drugs. Mama. It was merely a means of survival—a way to stop the pain in my head and the emptiness in my world. It was merely a way to embody the numbness. It was never for pleasure or for some great high. It was never a way to enjoy my world; it was merely a way to survive my world."

On Saturday, my son left for an overnight surfing trip with his friends. On Saturday, my mind was in a quiet place as I envisioned him in the water, riding the waves. and smiling as his life slowly returned to a good place. However, a series or chain of events prompted me to text him: *"Hey, sweet boy, I hope you're enjoying your weekend."* Second text: *"Remember you told me, as soon as you got to the campground, you would send a picture."* My third text message: *"Hey baby, where is Mama's cute picture?"*

Seven hours later, there still was no response. Seven hours later, my world stopped again, and I faded into the darkness—a place we go when the disease of addiction plays a role in our lives.

Finally, a response: *"Hey, Mama, sorry. I just saw your text. Give me a minute, and I will send you a picture."* Two more hours passed. No picture; no more text messages. It was now 11:45 p.m., and a strange text message appeared on my phone: *"Hey, can I spend the night at your house? Please, Mama?"*

*"Okay,"* was the only response my fingers could muster.

He arrived at 12:47 a.m. He sat on the couch and began to cry uncontrollably as the words formed out of his tears. "I hate this life, Mama. I hate my life." The words poured out of him like a river rushing in a storm, over and over and over. And so I did what any mother would do: I held him. I kissed his head, and I whispered, over and over and over, "I love you, baby. Mama is here." Slowly, he began to melt into my arms as he fell into a peaceful sleep. He looked so small, so fragile, so pale. All I could do was hold him and rock him back and forth and back and forth. I watched as he breathed in and out, until only the silence of the night could be heard.

I have no idea where he was for nearly twelve hours, and he would not say, so I stopped asking. I just enjoyed the time we shared on Sunday—a long drive into Long Beach (mostly without talking), a walk around the marina, an ice cream cone (mint chip, his favorite), followed by two hours reminiscing about his youth. As we began our long ride back home, he stared out the window, with just these few words spoken: "I wish I could just find a job and move here, Mama. I wish I could live in one of those apartments, alone, just once." This was followed by more silence and more sadness and darkness in his eyes. "I wish I could just be normal, just for one day. Just one day. Do you think God will ever let me have that?"

And so today, on Monday morning, when I woke up, I whispered to the universe, "Knock, knock. But there was no reply, so once again I whispered, Knock Knock ...

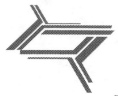

# Their Stories Live On

Giving back is an enormous part of survival, an enormous part of saying thank you to those who have stood by your side. Some of the stories that follow do not have a happy ending—they are told by parents who lost a child to the disease of addiction. Perhaps these stories can offer a reason to seek treatment or offer a better understanding of the journey on which the disease of addiction takes the entire family.

Other stories, though, are messages of hope, as told by those who made it through the maze of addiction—their stories are offered here to show you that there is survival. These stories express the strength and courage in taking the next step, entering a treatment program, and admitting you have a problem greater than yourself. When a person enters that door, he must walk a path that often breaks him down before it builds him back up, back to normal. This journey to survival is not easy path.

A heartfelt thank you to all who offered their stories, told of their struggles, and shared their triumphant journey back to clean.

Perhaps you will emerge with a greater understanding of the overwhelming pain and agonizing struggles that this terrible disease causes for its unsuspecting victims. Addiction is a disease, not a choice. No disease is ever a choice.

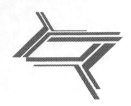

# My Story

### By Dean Ingram

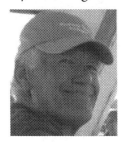

Alone (again) on my boat with an enormous amount of cocaine, I fully intended to explode my heart. Cutting fat lines sure to end my misery, an unrelenting voice in my head urgently insisted that I write this down. Finally giving in, I found a pen and began to write. My hand would not stop writing. What spilled out onto that paper astounded me to such a degree that I threw the cocaine overboard. Alive and 20 years later, those very words were the beginning Chapter in my own book "Dark to Light."

Mind you, my story is not unique, nor is it special. I'm just a fellow who started drinking at the age of twelve and grew up without the tools to grow up. I spent fifty-five years in trying, succeeding, pissing it all away, mental breakdowns, attempted suicides, multiple hospital stays, digging myself out, trying again, succeeding, and falling right back down that dark hole.

I was the perfect victim

To become that perfect victim, however, takes a lot of work. One must have a place to hide. One must have a partner so self-absorbed that one's behavior goes unnoticed—or ignored. One must have a steady supply of money to spend in bars. One must have a drug dealer who can be called at any hour to fulfill one's wants and needs. One must have a history of depression to fall back on, if ever questioned seriously about one's behavior. It would all add up to a very nicely wrapped package of pity.

Ah, the fuel of the victim; pity is like a salve. The bar is the perfect place for pity to flourish, or so it seemed. The fellow on the next bench may listen to every word I say, and he may acknowledge the very unfairness that brought me here. If I happen to buy him another beer, he'll listen all the more and nod his head knowingly as I tell my sad tale.

But over the course of six years, I fell deeper and deeper into the illusion that it really was everyone else's fault, and I had no blame. I wasn't hurting anyone. I was just going off by myself, minding my own business, because obviously, no one cared. Truth is; I am the only one who didn't care.

My last drink was Sunday night, Sept. 28, 2003. I had been listening to live music at the local tavern and enjoying myself. Upon driving myself home at 2:30 in the morning, I blacked out on a curve and woke with someone pounding on the window of my truck. "Are you all right? Are you all right?" I looked up and saw that my truck was in a ditch, head first. I quickly surmised that I could simply back out of this ditch and drive home. The fellow at my window thought this was a bad idea, but I could not be persuaded, so I followed through on my plan.

On waking up the next morning, I could remember only bits and pieces of the night before, and I finally realized—this has to stop. It was time for all of this to stop. I was miserable no matter what I did. If I drank, I was miserable. If I didn't drink, I was miserable. If I smoked pot, I was miserable. If I didn't, I was miserable. If I talked to anyone, I was miserable. If no one was there to talk to, I was miserable.

This went on for a week, at the end of which time my broken brain decided that I should go down to my boat. I should sail out to the middle of the Puget Sound, turn on the propane, light a match, and disappear into the mist. How romantic that would be! A statement. How could I be blamed?

I would be thanked for ending the misery that I had caused everyone. Finally, a practical solution with a fair chance of success! I had not seen success for quite some time, and the chance was seductive.

On the way to my boat that day, I passed a sign that read "Hospital," and for the briefest moment, I thought, *What if?* It was as if God's hand took the wheel, and I followed the sign. I drove to the emergency entrance, went to the front desk, and burst into tears. "I need help." I was still sobbing as they checked me into a psychiatric ward, where I stayed for three days.

On the fourth day, a meeting was held between the doctor, my wife, and me. The doctor told my wife that I was a late-stage alcoholic with liver damage, I was a drug addict, and I was clinically depressed. He expressed the difficulties ahead recovering from just one or two of these addictions, let alone all three. I remember the shocked look on my wife's face. Had she not realized what was going on with me all this time? … She left …

They signed me up for a twenty-eight-day alcohol recovery program at a local rehab facility, beginning my new and unrealized life. Somewhere during the second week in treatment, I noticed that some of my recovery associates were more cheerful and positive than I, and they seemed to be getting it. Some were even excited by the possibility of never having to drink again. I still wasn't ready to let go of that.

Then something unfamiliar happened; I raised my head, and I looked someone in the eye. I was amazed—he looked back, and we started a conversation. What did I want to get out of this? What did this person want to get out of this? The answers were slow to come. Over the remaining two weeks, the fact that those around me were actively seeking recovery finally convinced me that I could let go of the notion that I could do it all by myself. I realized that I had been fighting my entire life. I wasn't sure what I was fighting for anymore but still, I was fighting. It all seemed so silly.

Lying in my bunk one night, I finally decided just to let go and ask God for help. I had surrendered. I had acknowledged the first step in Alcoholics

Anonymous: We admit that we are powerless over alcohol, that our lives have become unmanageable. I felt relieved; I said the words out loud. I listened to the words as they bounced around in my head, and I thought, *My God, this might actually be possible after all.*

That was my turning point. It was the first time in a while that I began to believe something positive about myself. I came to understand that the idea of recovery is not to stop drinking; it is to learn how to live without alcohol. I am still an alcoholic; my goal is just to not act like one.

I am most grateful for the help I have received in the last ten years of my life. I am told that I have become a genuinely good person. Ten years ago, no one would have trusted me to walk their dog, but today … well, today I have the trust of those in my life that matter. I have responsibilities, and I am living up to those responsibilities.

Many other wonderful things have become possible through sobriety but for me. One of the most important things is being able to love unconditionally and to be able to receive love unconditionally, to the best of my understanding. Love is a self-fulfilling prophecy, as long as I just let it be. I don't judge; I don't expect; I don't resent; and I don't fool myself or my love, so today, I get to experience the gift of love.

Keep in mind that there are still days that I let down my guard and dwell in my head, but relief today comes from giving back to those who have suffered, much the same as I have. This is the honesty that saved me.

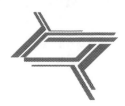

# TYLER'S STORY

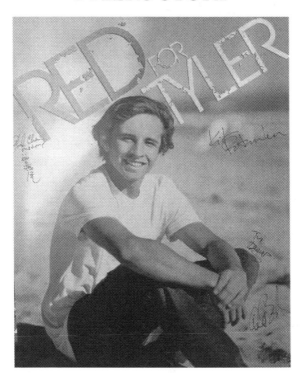

Tyler MacLeod (as offered by his loving Mother)
September 15, 1994–September 24, 2012

This is Tyler' Story – as Tyler would have wanted it told.

It was my senior year, and I was very excited to finish up my last year of high school. As a well-established senior, I was ready to conquer the year with my volleyball teammates and many other friends in my community.

A couple of weeks after school started I was walking to my car to get lunch at Panera with my friend Morgan. Morgan had been my best friend since fifth grade. We had a lot in common; we both lived in downtown Huntington Beach, and had lived there our whole life. Morgan has brown hair, brown eyes, and a laugh that makes you believe you're actually funny.

Morgan's sense of humor is the absolute best; the mix of immaturity and the fact that she is so relatable, makes her more entertaining than a dog on a skateboard. However, my favorite feature of my best friend is how much she cares about things, animals, people, causes; she puts everything and everyone ahead of her own needs.

That day (as told by Morgan) I was walking to my car after fourth period and was surprised to see friend Tyler MacLeod walking toward me—I hadn't seen him since eighth-grade graduation. Now, he was like a ghost; we almost couldn't tell if he was actually there or if we were just seeing things. He gave us a wink and a quick warm smile and said hello.

It wasn't until the next day that we all found out about Tyler. Tyler had been the most popular boy in school, possibly because of his athletic ability. Tyler played baseball, basketball, soccer, lacrosse and many other sports, and he surfed too. Maybe it was because his older brother, whom he idolized. also excelled in school, in soccer ... and picking up chicks. Maybe it was his ultra-involved PTA mom, who was everyone's favorite volunteer, or his successful realtor father, whose picture was on posters and open house signs throughout Huntington Beach. My personal opinion, though, is while all these factors helped to make him great, but Tyler was the most popular kid in school because he was known as a stand-up guy.

I had known Tyler since kindergarten, and we had been in class together many times. But in fifth grade, everything changed for me. I was the tall awkward girl with crooked teeth, and it didn't help that my mom let me wear jeans with patches. I had a flip phone, and an iPod, neither of which helped me combat the terrible insults the other kids hurled at me. I was a prime target for being bullied. They called me a giraffe and a horse, and those insults only made me more introverted. I had few friends and would play basketball with the boys in my spare time instead of skateboarding, surfing, or playing soccer, which were the popular activities in my beach community.

One day in PE, the substitute said we could hula-hoop or play football. Of course, all the boys wanted to play football, and all the girls wanted to hula-hoop—all the girls except for me. It was Tyler and another boy running the show, and when I looked like I wanted to play, Tyler was happy to include me unlike the other boys who looked confused, and thought, I couldn't compete.

Tyler said to me, "If you want to play, then you're in," and with that, I joined the game. It was as simple as that to Tyler. There were no stereotypes or prejudgments. I threw the football, and caught passes, and was able to prove them all wrong. I felt like I had just won the Super Bowl. I felt accepted and included, finally. Tyler was the one person who was a friend to me when no one else cared to be. I didn't go home crying and my depression lessened a little bit that day. That was one of the happiest memories I have of Tyler, he was my best friend and he changed my life.

Throughout middle school, Tyler continued to support me. We were both athletes, and we would always wave and talk at the sports awards when we could. Dwyer Middle School would be a turning point for us both, though. For me, middle school was an amazing time. I I finally grew into my tall stature, I filled out and got braces to fix my teeth. I started straightening my hair and choosing my own clothes, which proved beneficial for my social status.

For the first time in a long time, I had tons of friends and was very popular—I escaped being bullied, and the sadness that came with it. Middle school was great for Tyler, too; he had lots of friends and was the standout person on all of his teams. But slowly, I started to notice changes in Tyler's behavior and by eighth grade, he seemed a little more isolated. The kids said he was dealing pot or smoking pot. I did not know what to make of it; none of the other kids I knew were even thinking about it. Eighth-grade went by in a flash. The next year, Tyler was enrolled in a private high school called Mater Dei while the rest of us remained at Huntington Beach High School.

Tyler's parents must have wanted to remove him from his old friends, but of course he made new ones. Tyler made a lot of friends at Mater Dei, most of which I met my sophomore year in high school at a friends birthday party. There was Alex, Jianna, Misty, Ava and many of Tyler's middle school friends were there as well. That was a memorable night, and the commonality between all of us was that we all knew and loved Tyler.

At my varsity volleyball team pictures later that year, I heard the news about Tyler. I found out from my coaches, Craig Pazanti and Kendra, that Tyler Macleod had died. Shortly after his 18th birthday, Tyler had left this earth. I was in shock; I couldn't believe that it was true. Maybe they had the wrong name. I just couldn't believe that Tyler, my friend since elementary school was gone.

I drove my car home and parked behind my house, it suddenly hit me. I screamed, I cried, and I asked Tyler, "why he would do this to all the people who loved him?" Tyler's death was preventable; Tyler died of a heroin overdose.

The following week would prove to be one of the hardest times I would ever gone through. Kids were crying left and right; many needed to see the school counselors. The next day they started a Facebook group, and requested that everyone wear red to show their support and honor for Tyler. They also said that Tyler's mom, Nancy, would be at the football stadium the day after her son's death, just to see all of us wearing red for her son. The turnout was tremendous; it was like the whole community was wrapping their arms around Nancy. I think the most shocking part was seeing Nancy that the event. What a defining moment in her life that she could come to comfort us, even though it was her son that had just died.

The whole week would carry on like this, and the school soon turned red, and I mean red. Red on the trees, on the fences, on our clothing ... and in our hearts. I wore a red bow in my hair to every practice and every game that season. I cried all the time during volleyball. I was a mess and found myself tearing up as I drove home each day. We all noticed Tyler's empty desk, but we refused to take out of the classroom. The loss did not get easier as the days went on, and our community was not healing.

And we held a candlelight vigil. There was no doubt in my mind that I was going; I picked my friend Kelsy Henderson, whom I had known since the second grade. I dressed in a red beanie, my volleyball letterman's jacket, black jeans, and an inspired (red) shirt. I picked up beautiful flowers and bought fake candles. As we arrived at the beach, hundreds of adults and children were already there, all with somber expressions on their faces.

We walked pillows of sand towards an intimate circle, where Tyler's friends told stories about him. Each of us took a turn to stand in the middle of the circle and say something about our friend, Tyler. As we all spoke, the mood suddenly changed, and our hearts began to heal.

All the stories were breathtaking; there was the one from his best friend AJ or his first valentine Cassidy, or his brother, Kyle. After all the shared history it was time for each of us to put down our candles and approach the circle. Suddenly, the circle became much larger. There were rows and rows of people that loved Tyler just as much as I did. When I finally got up to the candles, my hands shook uncontrollably. I did not know what they were doing.

My friend Davis held my hand in comfort as we walked towards the candles. I had a hard time seeing through all of my tears. There were so many flowers, it was hard to find a space for me to put my flowers; I finally found a spot. I was embraced with arms of love; one of those hugs was from Nancy. As I was crying, she told me two words: "stay strong." I drove home trying to concentrate by talking about normal things with Kelsy.

But all we could talk about was how Tyler was one of the ten people that we had gone to school with since kindergarten, and how he would not be continuing with us. When I got home, I crawled into my mother's arms and cried and cried like I was in the fifth grade all over again.

Then came the most difficult event; the funeral. Again, it was requested that everyone wear red. The Funeral was held at First Christian Church in Huntington Beach. Throughout the service, I rested my head on my mother's shoulder and listened as people shared their personalized raps, songs, speeches, and frustration about what had happened. At the end of the funeral service, everyone signed our names on the coffin.

The next weeks were filled with events, like "Red for Tyler", wristband giveaways and fund-raisers. The red around our school had grown into a phenomenon that would promote drug awareness and prevention. It was amazing to see the progress; some kids were getting clean and were taking their futures more seriously because of Tyler. There were promos, seminars, and a video showing other people's struggle with addiction. Many volunteers worked the events with a smile. Everyone could purchase "Red for Tyler" shirts, stickers, and bracelets, and everyone did.

The months passed slowly after Tyler's death, but they passed. Classmates were accepted into their dream schools, and CIF championships were won. We ate bagels, and won sports championships, and failed Mr. Brown's econ final. Life went on after Tyler's death. At graduation, everyone realized how far we had come as a community. High school graduation was such a fulfilling time, but a lot of students did not want to graduate without Tyler.

Tyler was meant to graduate with us. He was meant to graduate with his lacrosse team, his prom date, his admirers, his friends, his teachers, and with the kids like me who had known him since kindergarten. We continued to ware our Red for Tyler bracelets and we kept posting Instagram photos and inviting friends to join the Facebook group in honor of Tyler. Tyler did graduate with all of us; he was in our heart and on our mind.

Tyler was not an empty desk in zero period, or an empty chair at our high school graduation. Tyler was the hero that helped me, and many others out of our depression, and isolation. Tyler's legacy continues to inspire other addicts, and many children and parents, and the world.

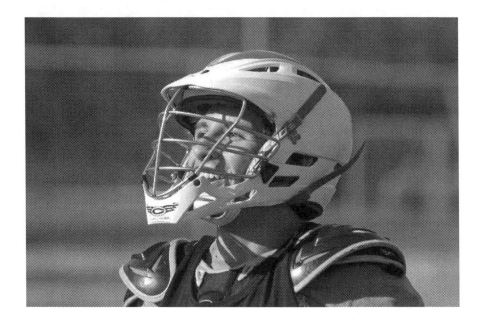

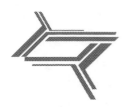

# ALEX'S STORY

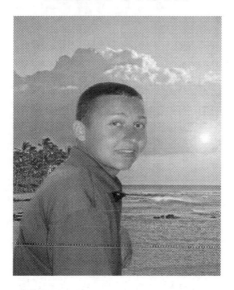

Alexander Joseph Marks (as offered my his loving Mother)
July 28, 1993–February 5, 2013

The death certificate from the Orange County coroner arrived in our mailbox; it read, "Cause of death: acute heroin intoxication."

On February 6, 2013, my husband found our nineteen-year-old son, Alex, dead in his room at our home in Huntington Beach, California. I was away on a business trip in Orlando, Florida. I cannot put into words, the feeling a parent feels, flying home alone knowing, your child was already gone. It is indescribable. My husband told me he found a needle and heroin on Alex's desk. I could not believe that my son had turned to heroin; we were devastated to learn this was the way our son had died.

The wound was—and still is—so deep, so raw; we thought he'd overcome addiction. We thought he was doing well, working during his college break, and would go back to school to become an electrician. Externally that is what we thought, but now we understand that inside, he was so sick ... there was no note. He accidentally overdosed because he had not built up a tolerance to the amount he ingested. After so many months of being clean, he used too much too fast. We do not know the answers to the whys, and the what-ifs that constantly swirl through our minds.

During elementary and junior high school years, Alex had been bullied. He had two rare medical conditions—osteochondromatosis, a rare bone disease; and Von Willebrand disease, a blood-clotting disorder—in addition to mental health issues. He had experienced much more than any kid should at such a young age—many surgeries, doctor visits, and home health-care nurses administrating IV medication. In or around the fifth grade, Alex was diagnosed with ADHD.

Then, in his freshman year of high school, his grandma died and he turned to pot and alcohol, which led to pills and other drugs. His grandma had been the rock in his life; he did not want to live without her. He had a rough time in high school. He didn't have a girlfriend, so he didn't attend high school dances, and he wasn't involved in activities. He didn't have true friends, good friends. Alex was not involved activities, no matter how many times we encouraged him to get involved; what he had, were other teens that used him.

Alex self-medicated to cover his pain. When his addiction progressed, we had him admitted to the University of California, Irvine, as well as Loma Linda Medical Center psychiatric hospital. Upon release, he attended a thirty-day local treatment program at Chapman House in Orange, California. He sought help from many medical professionals and was diagnosed with depression and bipolar disorder. Nothing we tried, however, seemed to help him. We sent Alex away to Heritage Residential Treatment Center in Provo, Utah, where he spent eight months in treatment.

He came home, graduated high school, and within a few months, he was back to hanging out with the "drug friends" and local teens he'd met at Heritage Center. In December 2011, at the age of eighteen, Alex was arrested and charged with a felony—receiving stolen property with the intent to sell. He was sent to jail for seven months.

Alex followed the path of many before him. He was stealing for drug money, for Oxycontin. He was sentenced to three years' probation, with the stipulation that if he completed all that was required, the felony would be removed from his record. These tough learning experiences made him realize he never wanted to go back to jail. He wanted his freedom. He wanted his life back.

On July 5, 2012, Alex was released from jail at 3:00 a.m. (without guidance, without supervision—something I will never understand). Alex was determined to do what he needed to be do—see his probation officer and attend weekly drug classes. He was overwhelmed with the court fees and the classes he had to take, but he was willing to comply in order to gain his freedom.

The price was high, and hanging over his head was the thought of how he could pay all the money he was required to pay and attend all the necessary meetings when he didn't have a car. He quickly learned the OCTA bus schedule and got where he needed to be on time. Each time that he was drug tested, he tested clean.

My Alex was once again a joy to be around; he had a few ups and downs, but all in all, we believed the worst was over. He started an electrician program at Long Beach City College and never missed a day that entire semester. He registered for the next semester and was on the right track—or so we thought.

On Tuesday, February 5, 2013, two young adults came to the house. We believe Alex may have met these "friends" at his court-ordered drug classes. We also believe Alex purchased heroin that day from these "friends." Alex returned home from meeting with his probation officer around 7:30 p.m. He had some soup, watched the Lakers game with his dad and his dog, Charlie, and then said, "Good night. I love you" and went to his room. At approximately 5:30 a.m. on February 6, 2013, my husband found Alex in his room. He was dead. The coroner's report stated Alex had died at approximately midnight on February 5.

I'm sure this story is all too similar to many stories you've heard or read. This story has been told (to some degree), by other families who have been through this same nightmare. This ordeal has been the most difficult four and a half years of our lives, but I have a passion to keep my son's memory alive. Alex loved cooking, eating, and gardening, and he loved his dog and his family. We asked that all donations for Alex go to the Huntington Beach Dog Beach, where he loved to take his dog "Charlie.

One of the most frustrating parts of this journey was how difficult it was to get good help for our son. There was no place for him to go where he could meet and associate with good people—people who would mentor him and others like him. I prayed each and every day for God to shine his light upon Alex, to bring the right people into his life. He needed someone other than his parents to help him ... but this did not happen. My heart aches for the many teens that leave this world because of addiction. They simply feel powerless to stop the power of drugs.

I see the pain that our entire family has endured; even Alex's beloved dog, Charlie, is sad. There is no room for me in my owner's life, because my owner, Alex, my best friend, is gone.

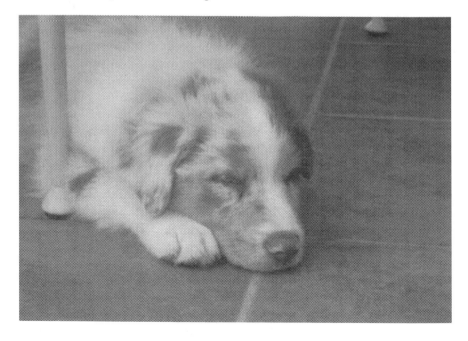

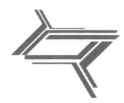

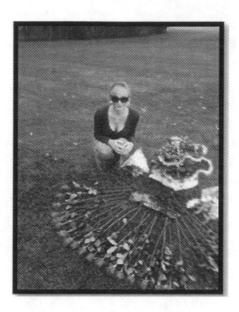

**Late last year Taylor died alone of a drug overdose at the tender age of nineteen.**

Taylor was the love of my life, with his sweet blue eyes, blond wavy hair, and his warm, beautiful smile. He had a unique, gregarious personality and had many friends. I won't forget the day my husband told me that Taylor had died.

The world went silent for me. My knees buckled, my mind raced, and my heart broke into a million pieces. There was a deep pain in my stomach on the ride home with my husband. The world stood silent as the tears ran down my face. In the hours that followed, my devastation turned into denial. I was in a state of shock. I felt this was a cruel joke, that a mistake had been made. My soul cried out for Taylor as the slideshow of our life danced through my mind. I didn't sleep that night or for many nights thereafter. The following day, I awoke to a new world, a new life, one without my beautiful boy, my son.

As I gazed out the window from my home in Laguna Beach, the ocean was still, as were my emotions. I questioned the existence of a higher power. I could not see or feel Taylor, and I could not feel the presence of God. I was numb. Flowers arrived, but I couldn't look at them. I didn't open the cards until a week later; most of the flowers had withered and died, as if they were mourning with me.

For the past ten years, I had been working for a Christian treatment center as a crisis counselor. I had helped hundreds of families, nationwide, get help for their loved ones' addictions. I had coached them, cried with them, and celebrated their victories. I was good at my job and very dedicated to the families I was privileged to know. I knew of many who were once lost but found a new life, free from addiction. I had seen the hand of God move miraculously in their lives. Families were reunited, and marriages were restored, with gratitude and hope on the horizon.

The other side of that coin was that I had witnessed and heard about death far too often. I was the great consoler, standing shoulder-to-shoulder with families who had lost their son or daughter to addiction. Like any other mother, I thought death only happened to other people.

For years, we sent Taylor to wilderness camps, military schools, and many different treatment facilities. Taylor knew God. He had heard and learned about sobriety and how bad drugs were. All the knowledge in the world, however, could not keep Taylor from doing what he loved—getting high. There are times I have blamed myself, blamed his father, and blamed treatment centers, but it has been hard for me to blame Taylor. It seemed that hundreds of his friends attended his funeral. My veil hid my tears as I laid my son to rest. I really could not tell you what was said at the funeral service or who was there. I tried to smile and thank the guests, but this was now my cross to bear. Taylor's death became my reality. I stayed in shock and denial for a long time.

My husband has been in the addiction-treatment industry for the past fifteen years. He was supportive, loving, and caring during this difficult time. My husband loves me very much and cared deeply for Taylor. He approached me with the concept of opening our own treatment center, one that Taylor would have liked and where he could have overcome his addiction. I decided to leave my job of ten years to pursue the mission of honoring my son and helping others.

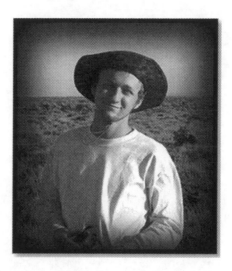

It was not long after I had stopped working and slowed down a bit that reality set in. Taylor was dead. He died and is not coming back. All the emotions that I had held back came to the surface, and I would cry uncontrollably. I needed that time. I needed to grieve and acknowledge my loss. I was angry with God. I was angry with myself. I was angry with Taylor. Nothing was going to bring him back.

This is the hard truth that I have had to accept. It is not easy. I wonder what I could have done differently.

May God bless you,
**Nicole Browne – A Mothers Mission**

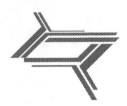

# CHRIS LOVE'S STORY

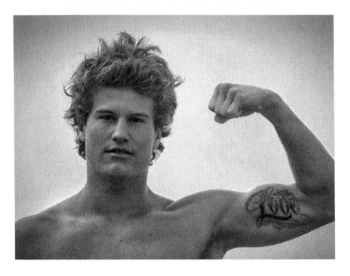

**W**here does a mother begin?

I was having one of the best nights of my life. I was out with the two men in my life, my two sons, also known as two of the four lights of my life; my oldest son Jason and my youngest son Chris. We went to a movie together …

We spent a wonderful evening together laughing playing around, and just having a great time together. How does a mother, whose children are her *everything*, go from that, to the very next day being the very worst day of her life? Life can change that fast—in an instant—for any of us.

The next day, after such an incredible evening of fun, I received the most dreaded news a mother could ever hear. My daughter had to tell me that her younger brother, my youngest child, my son Chris, had passed away. My whole world came crashing down on me. I was in a state of disbelief, a state of shock. How could this be? How could this possibly be? Chris was only twenty. He was still my little boy, my baby.

Chris had dabbled in smoking pot. He had a medical marijuana card, that he received from a doctor for his ADHD. He was also on prescription Xanax for anxiety. Chris was trying to cope with the stress from his father's illness as well. Two weeks before his passing, Chris turned himself into the courts and asked for jail time. He needed to get clean. He told me, "Mom, I don't want to live this way anymore. I want to get off all these drugs."

Chris got out of jail a few days before he passed away. I remember he had a bad toothache and went to the dentist, where they did a "couple" of root canals. The dentist gave him hydrocodone; 7.5 mg. for the pain.

On that last night, he went out with a friend after the movie ended, and he received news that his dad's illness was not going well. Chris's friend said Chris was so distraught, he decided to call up an old friend he'd met at a Narcotics Anonymous program. He left that friend and went over to an old friends house, and she gave him heroin.

Hours later, Chris was having trouble breathing; she called a friend of Chris, whose Mother said, "call 911." She didn't want to get busted, so she chose not to call 911 for several more hours. By the time she called, it was too late, my son, my beautiful child, my youngest, was gone.

What do you tell kids when they think of trying drugs, even if they say "it's only pot"? How do you get through to someone? *Don't* do it. Just don't start! They think they're just having fun and that they can control it. How do you tell someone, "It will take over your life"? How can you make them understand, "It will take everything from you until there is no more to take, except your life"? How do you tell them?

How do you tell someone, "If you do this, you not only will harm yourself, but you will destroy your family as well"?

None of us is guaranteed that tomorrow will come, but losing my son was something I never could have imagined. It's an unfathomable pain that no parent should ever have to go through, and the pain never goes away. *Never* !

Forever Chris Love's mother,
Melody

"I give all the credit to God for still being here. It is only through my faith in God that He has given me the strength to get through each day, and to know I will see my son again in Heaven one day! My love for my other children and grandchildren also keeps me going every day."

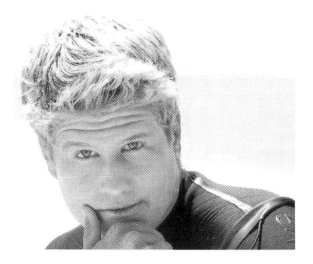

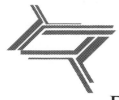

# Dimitri Zarate's Story

I first met Dimitri Zarate in 2010; he and my son were in a treatment center together. In June 2014, our paths crossed again. I had the immense pleasure to witness Dimitri's graduation from Drug Court, upon which his very well-earned new life was about to commence.

**What is Drug Court, and how does Drug Court work?**
Eligible drug-addicted persons may be sent to Drug Court in lieu of traditional justice-system case processing. Drug Court keeps individuals in treatment long enough for it to work, while supervising them closely.

For a minimum term of one year, participants are provided with intensive treatment and other services they require to get and stay clean and sober. Participants are held accountable by the Drug Court judge for meeting their obligations to the court, society, themselves, and to their families. They are regularly and randomly tested for drug use; required to appear in court frequently, so that the judge may review their progress; and rewarded for doing well or sanctioned when they do not live up to their obligations.

When I asked Dimitri to share his story of survival, he responded, "What should I say that might help someone reading my story"? I simply replied, "Allow me to print your graduation speech; it tells the entire story."

It is not often we are blessed to see the raw reality of survival when the disease of addiction is in the picture. However, it is only through our sharing of such gripping stories, that we can begin to offer hope to someone in need of such a miracle. Perhaps Dimitri's story will be that miracle to someone in need.

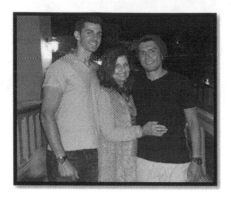

Dimitri Zarate's Drug Court Graduation Speech

"Religion is for people who want to stay out of hell; spirituality it is for those who have been to hell."

There are numerous sayings that I have come across through my countless attempts at getting sober, and that one resonates with me today. In active addiction, my hopelessness was so deep that death seemed like the only way out of my private hell. How many more times was I going to have to go through the loop? Was nineteen times enough? How many more rehabs could I go to? Was seven enough? How many more overdoses and seizures could my body handle? Was eleven enough? I eventually planned my suicide, because I didn't have an answer to those questions. I felt that there was no other way out of that living hell.

**Ladies and gentlemen, welcome to my spiritual bottom.**

On February 6, 2012, the culmination of over fifteen years of drug dependence had landed me into a dire situation, where I had a decision to make. I had to decide if I was going to change my life or die an addict's death. I had been assessed for Drug Court in the past, but in my heart, I knew I wasn't ready, and so I declined the program. But when the wreckage of eleven court cases and fourteen felonies were sending me to prison, I had an honest conversation with Lorrie. As she walked away from the "cage" and looked back over her shoulder at me, she asked one simple question: "Do you want our help or not?" Homeless, alone, and a frail frame of a man riddled with track marks, I clung to the cage as I looked at her and said, "Yes."

**I welcome you all to my legal bottom.**

As I look back, I feel that day was the beginning of what the Big Book of Alcoholics Anonymous describes as a "spiritual" experience or a "personality change" that is sufficient to bring about recovery. I was given the gift of desperation that day and the willingness to try it someone else's way. I was out of ideas.

I don't plan on describing in detail, my history, because it is just that—history. What I will tell you is this: I was raised in a loving family and always had what I needed when I was growing up. Addiction doesn't discriminate; it tore through my life and everyone's life around me for far too long. I feel it is important that I mention something, as it is the most significant part of my story: four months into my jail sentence, on May 5, 2012, I was hit with the worst experience of my life. My brother had to perform a duty that no person should ever have to perform. He had to visit his brother in jail and tell him that our sister, who was diagnosed with leukemia a month earlier, had abruptly passed away.

I vividly remember that day and leaving the visiting area to be alone with myself, and my consequences. Alone. I never got to say good-bye to my sister; I had to listen to her funeral on a payphone in the bowels of Theo Lacy Jail. Alone.

**Welcome to my emotional bottom.**

My intention is not to bring down those in the courtroom, as this is a day of celebration. I have never been a fan of focusing on myself or having other people focus on or honor me. I didn't even bother to walk the path at my college graduation. But today is the most significant accomplishment of my life. Today is a victory for me. I never thought I would make it out of that hell, nor would I have the ability to deal with the Mount Everest of wreckage that was waiting for me upon my release. Today, I want to give hope to the hopeless, because there is a way out.

Today, my life is amazing. Long gone are the days of rotting away in a dark room by myself with a needle in my arm—a glance around the room today is evidence of that. On the day I was arrested, the only people in my life were three family members who didn't even want to talk to me. Today, I had to request a larger courtroom to fit just a portion of the amazing people I have in my life.

I can't thank you all for what you have done for me; I have been given the gift of so many rich and authentic relationships, and today, my life is so full. I have been able to accomplish more than I could have imagined in the past two years. Toward the end of my six-month treatment at Gerry House, I began taking the bus from Santa Ana to Saddleback College to begin the certification program in alcohol and drug studies to become a counselor. I completed my final internship and graduated that two-year program with a 4.0 grade point average.

For the past year, I have been working as a case manager at a center for addiction treatment, where I was voted Employee of the Month for the first time in my life. I truly feel I have found my calling and a passion for helping others. I am blessed to begin the next chapter of my professional career with an amazing new team. I no longer have to take the bus, because I also completed my eighteen-month DUI course; today, I have my license back—and a car.

The material things in life are nice, but nothing is more valuable than being a man of integrity. Today, I have the ability to look at life with a healthy perception, and today, I have hope for the future.

Today, my options are endless, and I have so many choices; the right choices are open to me. For so long, I had no choice but to use. For all these things, I am forever grateful to the Drug Court team for keeping me on track. I owe my life to all of you.

Thank you for looking at me and seeing a man, not a case number. My sessions with you came at just the right time. Thank you for putting the fear of God in me on a daily basis, which always kept me on the path that

I needed to be on. But I do look forward to having my blood pressure return to normal.

Overall, my experience in Drug Court has taught me three priceless life principles that I will take with me for the rest of my life; these principles are indispensable. They are humility, accountability, and responsibility. So many other people have been an integral part of my life, and I sincerely thank you all from the bottom of my heart. I do want to thank a few people in particular, though.

To my brother, you have shown me what strength looks like and how an honorable man should behave. Jason, I have the utmost respect for you and I thank you for your endless support.

To my mom, only you and I know the personal hell that this has been. I know we have had our struggles over the years, but thank you for always believing in me and never giving up hope.

To my beautiful sister, Lisette, I miss you more and more every day. I wish that you were here today to see that your only wish for me is finally coming true. Sis, I am finally doing it.

To all my peers in Drug Court, I leave you with a quote from Coach Vince Lombardi. "The greatest accomplishment is not in never falling but in rising again after you fall."

*I thank you all for my 857 days of sobriety.*
—Dimitri Zarate

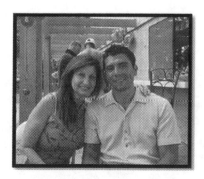

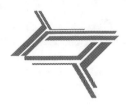

# A LETTER TO MY SON

By Trisha

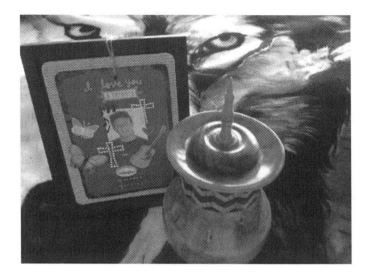

Son, you were taken without warning, leaving a wake of heartache behind. There is no looking back, there is only looking back. I can't negotiate a deal for one more conversation, because you slipped off the edge where you so often spent time. You waited for the angel of life or the angel of death to deliver release. We know which one came. There are no more chances to get it right. Twenty-six years sounds like a lot, but it wasn't enough. No amount of time is enough to say, "*I can now live without you*" or that "*I'm ready to be childless.*"

You are gone, and I ache. I want more time, but I'll never be granted another minute. I had no control over how, when, or why you died. In the end, I was powerless. I helped you stay alive for a while, but I wasn't able to help you in the early hours of June 11. Regret won't budge the circumstances. The force of my "want" can't amend a moment, the moment you died.

I was blessed that you were my child. Even after drugs took you and changed you, not once did I give up on you. Don't give up on me. Lend me your life force and help me move on. There's nothing left for me but to get on with grieving and count up my loss. Nothing will get you back. The space that you once filled is with me all the time; a hole the shape of you. It gets so big some days that I can't see or feel anything else. The reflections of a mourner are a relentless accounting, especially when the loss is sudden, shocking, and out of sequence. The future I was counting on has vaporized. My hope is that one day soon I can live in gratitude for the time that we had. We had some good times, you and me. For some, it is hard to speak of you; for me, it is hard not to, son.

Love,
Mommy

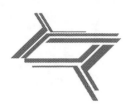

# Brent Jason

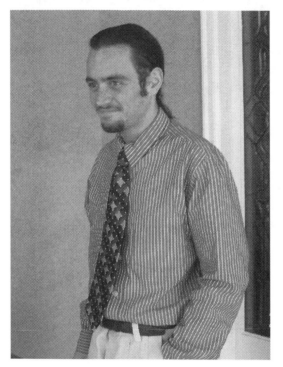

**Part of Our Hearts Forever**

Could we ever forget your sparkling eyes or the way
you brightened each day, or your smile which is etched
in our memories, so you're never far away.

Could we ever forget those priceless moments?
The answer, of course, is never. For you were part of our lives for a
brief time, but you'll be part of our hearts forever. So completely
you were here among us, and so quickly you were gone.
High on angels' wings you rise.
Onward, upward to heavenly skies.
Where are the words we long to say?

The words: they do not come.
To express our love and ease our pain,
so that we may begin to heal and look for joy again.

I will see you in our eternal life, my loving son!
Mom
xoxo

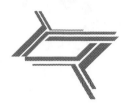

# THIS IS MY STORY

By Donald Keith

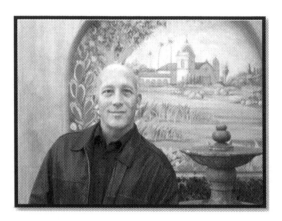

I was raised in a single-parent household in Anaheim, California. It was my mother, my sister, my brother, and me. Mom and Dad separated before I was born. I saw my dad every other weekend.

I was a very girly little boy, growing up in an ultra-conservative home. I instinctively felt different; as far back as I can remember. I should add that my father was very heavy-handed, and my sister, who was ten years older than I, frequently beat the hell out of me; she learned this behavior from my dad.

I am now aware of my first "addiction"—seeking approval. I learned early on what I had to do to get it, and I obsessed on it. It didn't matter what I thought; I was only focused on what I thought others thought of me. I made a conscious choice to "act" normal; I did not want to attract undue attention to me.

I knew that "normal" boys asked for a football at Christmas time, not an Easy Bake oven (which I truly wanted). I played Little League, Pop

Warner football, and soccer, just like a normal boy did. I was desperate to be a perfect child. There were kids who called me a "little girl" or "faggot," and that reminded me more and more that my truth, could never be known. I went to high school, where I continued on my path of the perfect "straight" life, even dating women. I began drinking at sixteen years of age—three or four beers here and there, nothing too crazy.

When I eventually came out to my mom when I was twenty-three, she vomited on me and asked me to move out. I went out that night and got drunk. It was my only coping skill at the time. After all, what else do you do when you mother says, "I wish you weren't my son."

I had been hired at the local Probation Department to work with minors in juvenile hall. I was so proud of that job. In the next handful of years, my drinking and drugging increased exponentially.

I went years without much contact with my family—my head told me that they hated me—so I found a new family among my friends. I was a regular at local gay clubs. For as much as I drank and used drugs, I never really had a taste for it, but I loved the "numb." I loved that I didn't have to feel very much. In 1993, I found my way to meth. It was true love. I lost a great deal of weight, which in my mind made me attractive to other guys. I thought I finally fit in; the party was on. I resigned from the Probation Department in 1994 and went on a five-year run. I spent my $12,000 retirement from the Probation Department in seven months, with nothing left to show for it.

My drinking and drugging became a daily habit, and I did whatever I had to do in order to have enough drug money. For someone who so desperately wanted to be "perfect," I had become the exact opposite. In my head, I was a victim. My family hated me; I had withstood my fair share of verbal and physical abuse, and I chose to carry the emotional baggage that had been handed to me during my childhood. Playing the victim allowed me to avoid any responsibility for my life. It was everyone else's fault.

In 1999, I was pulled over for a burned-out headlight, I was high, and the cop knew it immediately. I was arrested and placed on probation at the very same Probation Department where I had worked for six years. Slightly humbling experience. I was offered a court-ordered program in lieu of two years in prison. I accepted that program with no real intention of getting or staying clean. I began my journey in recovery—therapy, groups, 12-step meetings, and living in sober living. I graduated the program after fifteen months.

Shortly after graduating the program, I got a call from a local hospital; my mother had suffered a stroke. I went to the hospital to see my mom, with whom I had barely spoken in five years. My mother asked me to move in with her and help her as she recovered. At my sponsor's direction, I did just that. He told me to go and just be her son.

We had fifteen months together, and we learned to listen to one another. I changed her diaper, and I cooked for her. I drove her to her doctor's appointments, and I shopped for groceries. In recovery, I got to become the son that my mom deserved.

My mom was a huge fan of the Los Angeles Angels, and I surprised her with tickets to the Mother's Day celebration at Angels Stadium. She was beside herself with excitement. She had her Angels hat and Angels jacket, her Rally Monkey (the unofficial mascot for the Angels), and her thunder sticks—it was beautiful!

Shortly thereafter, she moved to Montana to be near my brother. Two months later, my brother called to tell me that the doctor had given Mom just a few days to live—her kidneys were shutting down.

I wanted to drink, I wanted to use, but I joined my sponsor at our usual 12-step meeting, where I shared, and I cried as I told everyone that I had no money to travel to Montana. I was living paycheck to paycheck. After the meeting, a group of friends told me they had taken up a collection during the break, and they handed me an envelope full of money, saying, "Go be with your mom."

I got to Montana, and I got to have that talk with my mom. She asked me to put my sobriety chip in the pocket of her robe. When I asked her why, she said, "I want to take it up and show your grandma." I got to hold her hand, just as she had done for me countless times. She passed a few days later.

The next year, as Mother's Day approached, my friends told me that they had bought tickets to the Mother's Day celebration at Angels Stadium to honor my mom. We went to the game, but before the game began, we went out to the center field fountain. We said a prayer, and then I poured a small amount of my mom's ashes into the fountain. She was such an Angels fan, and now, when the fountain shoots up in the air, my angel is in the outfield, and she continues to watch over me.

Eventually, I went back to college, and I now work as a clinician for the very same program from which I graduated many years ago. I still have a sponsor, I have my regular meetings, and I have a wonderful support group of friends. More important, today, I have hope.

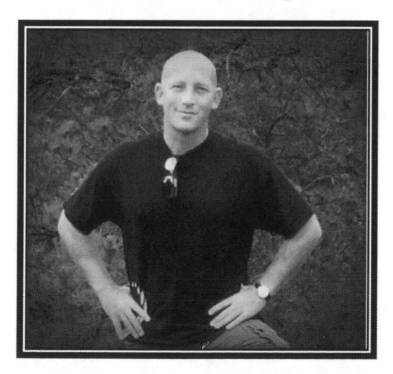

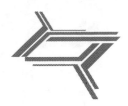

# TEMPTATION 7

Written by Tyler
On 6/1/2011
(A journal entry, shared by Tyler's mother, Janice)

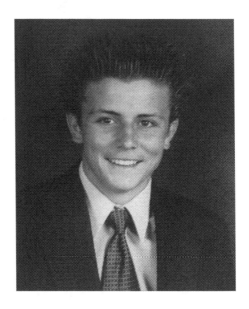

Eve: Write the story you would tell your children about your temptations and what happened as a result (read Genesis 2:3)

*05/21/1986 – 03/18/2012*

Dear children,
My temptations have put me in a world of hurt. They have lead to nothing but destruction and total mayhem. My temptations not have only hurt myself but have hurt many others as well. They did not just hurt many others but hurt the ones that love me most. They have stripped me naked and now, with the help of the Lord, who is clothing me, step by step.
Tyler

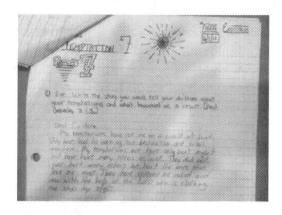

*Genesis 2:3*

**2** Thus the heavens and the earth were completed in all their vast array.
By the seventh day God had finished the work he had been
doing; so on the seventh day He rested from all His work. **3** Then
God blessed the seventh day and made it holy, because on it
He rested from all the work of creating that He had done.
—Genesis 2:2–3

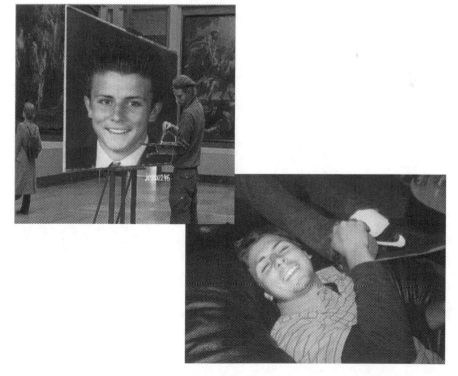

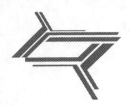

# LANCE HENRY
# THOMAS'S STORY

A beautiful young man, currently residing in California State Prison, sent the next story to me. This young man's story will touch your heart, bring tears to your eyes, and make you want to stand up and scream at what addiction has done to his life.

There is nothing about the disease of addiction that is glamorous or, in the writer's words, "cool." There is nothing that is worth the price you will pay. Your life, your soul, your friends, and your family become part of the drama that addiction brings to the table. Nobody wins; everybody loses.

I

MY NAME IS LANCE HENRY THOMAS. I was BORN IN SAN DIEGO
CA. ON January 3rd 1988. WHich would make me 26 years old
aS of Right Now. I've Spent the last 4 years of my life IN A
CaliForNia STATE PRISON Due To Some Bad DecisioNS And Misdirections.
IN MY Young adult life But it hasn't always Been like this I've
Seen life From Both Sides of the Spectrum.
     I was Born Into a Broken Family A Mother I'll JuSt label AS
"F" was a Rich kid With Daddy'S money who threw it all away for
drugs. ME Being the 1St BoRN was SuBJect to an intoxicated Birth
due to the Fact of her Being oN Drugs during pregnancy. MY Father I'll
Just label him as "T" was A outstanding athlete and a Scholar But
held Back by an alcohol problem and a new eScape Which was woRking.
"F" & "T" Never were Married had kids out of wedlock and I dont
Believe either of them were Ready for kidS. AT A Young age Id say
about 5 months old I had medical ComplicationS and needed Emergency
Surgery to Save my life. They took out 3 inches of my Intestine out But
NoT Before it killed me on the operating table. "CHildREN's HoSpital" in
San Diego Saved my life Brought me back on the table But put me in A CoMA.
I Remaind that way for a Few monthS at 7 months old I was
diagnoSed Type I diabetic and given a liFe expectancy of only 7 years.
MY Father "T" told them that his SoN was gonna make it through any
Hurdle life could present. I'll tell you my Early childhood presented
many HurdleS. But ONLY The Strong Survive. AT THE Age of 3 With
MY Mom "F" Still Batteling drug addiction was traveling With me in the
Front Seat of her Car With No CAR Seat and lost Control which made
her crash into a Fire Hydrant. I SubSequently Flew into the Front
WindShield. "F" Fled the Scene on Foot leaving me There for the
ParamedicS to Find ME. WHEN I was older I Found out From "T" that
She Fled the Scene and left me THERE Because she was High on METH &

& HeroIN and Feared going to Jail I guess Risking my life was not that Big of a deal. AT This point My Dad "T" had come to claim me From Polinski Child abuse center. MY Father later Got Full Custody of me and my Siblings due to the fact my mother Showed up to our Custody Court date Drunk & High and got kicked out of the Court Room. I havent Seen my mom since I was 3. I dont even Remember what she looks like. MY Father took Full Custody of us. I owe him my life even though he worked outrageous Hours and when he was home he drank obsessivly he kept me alive and he kept Food ON THE Table And A Roof over our head. ARound the Age of 4 My Father got Remarried to A lady She had two kids. I'll label her as "J". I wont go Into to much detail but From the age of 5 to the Age of 12 I was Subject to large amounts of torture and Abuse and cruelty. Not to Mention the kind of Company this lady who was married to my Dad Brought around. I can Remember drug use From "J" I can remember guys that were not my dad There a lot. IN oRder to keep my Brother & Sister Safe I took the Brunt of what ill Call Hurricane "J". Like I Said I wont go into too much detail But ill give you a couple of examples of the things She put me through. I Remember one time we lived in Vegas I had done my chores and I went to my Room to get away. "J"'s "Daughter I'll call her "J 2" Stormed in my Room and Said "look your gonna do my chores;", I told her "No that's why There You're Chores There for you to do." She told me "is that Right". Then she Stormed oFF. Next thing I know "J" and "J 2" Come in Slam open the door "J" Grabs my legs "J 2" grabs my arms they drag me down the Stairs and I Break Free by the kitchen "J 2" tackels me and knocks the wind out of me and then Kicks me in the Stomach. "J" & "J 2" Jie me up with an extension cord to bound me and throw Me in the Family Van and "J" Says "You think Your Slick Now You're

2

Never gonna see your dad again". I dont know where they were gonna take me but I Broke Free Kicked the door open and RAN Away My Dad Came And found me later and She made up some story to tell my Dad So all the negative was on me. I would get slapped and punched for no reason. It got so bad one time I had to miss a week of school due to Bruising. My Dad never Caught oN Because he would get off of work at 1AM or 2AM then Be back at 6:30AM that's the work hours remodeling the MGM Grand Called for So I was asleep when he came in and left for work. I can remember getting punched so hard and Bleeding just lying there thinking I wish I Could just die this pain is too much. But I never did I couldn't For my little Brother and sister. But the turmoil at home made me excel in other aspects of my life. Most kids when put through stuff like this Rebel and Cause problems. Instead I was great in school and great in Sports I had a natural gift for Baseball AND School. My Dad always Kept me in Baseball. He himself played ~~for the~~ for the Cardinals in the late 70's But he got hurt and lost that. Baseball and school was my life. IN 5th grade I was in G.A.T.E. classes and was class president and also playing on allstar teams and a number of travel Baseball teams. Such as the "Bulldogs" out of San Diego and the "Wave" out of San Clemente With them I got to play in Cooperstown classic and won. which made scouts for the ~~Jev~~ Junior olympic team Check me out. BY THIS TIME I was in middle school. My 5th Grade year "J" went to hit me and Instead of Being Scared I stood up to her as I was taller now And I hit her with a Broom and told my Siblings to run and I hit her again and Knocked her out and RAN. MY DAd foundout She was abusing me Cause I had bruising on my Face and he seen it. He divorced her. She Drained My Dads Bank accounts Broke the Windows out in our house

And my Dad's truck stole a lot of our stuff But she was gone. She left us struggeling we lived off Spagehtti o's and Ramen noodles for a year and at times didn't have enough money to buy my diabetic insulin. But we still had a home. She got my dad in trouble with the IRS But everything would work out in the end. Most Kids would Rebel Instead I thrived. I stayed far away from drugs because I hated what they had already taken from me By the 6th grade I was in "Avid" it was an Honor program in middle school and By 7th & 8th grade I was already taking high school courses. I Played on A winter ball team IN 8th grade For the high school I was gonna be going to the Following Year. And when I hit 9th grade I was already a starting 3rd baseman For Varsity baseball we won CIF Championships My 1st 2 years and also my 1st 2 years of Varsity football too. I had 4 Rings already I was done with my high school credits By my Sophomore year So I Just Breezed through stayed around to play football and Baseball and took cooking classes and teachers aid in The Library. My Junior year things Started happening for me I had a few Colleges after me for Baseball ONE Being SDSU. And the second being Cal State Fullerton. And A few Colleges Interested in me for my Academics. One Being Barry University out of Florida. They wanted me to work with them in Marine Biology In Partnership with the "EPA". And "UCSB" also because I was Interning at Scripps School of Oceanography in La Jolla, CA. Which partnerd with "UCSD". They gave me a Refrence to use for one of those Schools. My (SAT) Score was 1960 out of 2400 and my total "GPA" in all my 4 years of High School was 3.6. My Senior year I began to try Alcohol and I smoked a little Pot like all teens do. But The after baseball Season

3

towards the end of my Senior year my Brother after having his license only 1 month crashed his car into a tree going 70 MPH. He was only 30 seconds away from where we lived. I was told that Somebody in a Yellow Mustang Ran him off the Road And didn't even Stop to see if he was alright. What's crazy about that is that I was Supposed to go to work with him that night. I was Supposed to be in that car with him. But I ditched him and went to A party Instead. I'll Never forgive myself for that ever! After all those years of protecting him all the Sudden I couldnt protect him Anymore. He was gone. I Rememberd we ditched School that day And went to IN & out to get Burgers and I told him "Hey Dude, I love you man". And He told me "Dont go getting all gay on me Dude","I know you love me". That was the last time that happend between us. I had 2 voicemails when I Charged my phone the next day from him Right Before the crash. When I got home the next day my dad was there he said "LANCE Sit DOWN" Everybody was upset. I said Were's "my Brother" I've Been calling him all morning from my friends house phone that Dumbass HaHa". My Dad looked at me and said "LANCE he's Dead, He got IN A Crash lastnight" I didn't Believe it At First. I had another new Stepmom at the time she was a Cruel lady she told me to quit crying and man up I chased her down and threw a chair at her. She locked herself in her Room for awhile. I lost it I started doing every drug possible and drinking I had a Scholarship to Cal State Fullerton at this point. well I ended up taking so many drugs that I went blind for a couple of hours And had a minor stroke Because my diabeties was all messed up. I got out of the hospital a day Before my prom and the Same day as my prom was the Same day as my Brothers Funeral I'll always Remember that. Well Not soon after I graduated

I caught a case for possesion of Drugs and being high while driving. My 1st time in trouble. Then I lost my scholarship And my shot to play DiViSiON 1 Baseball in College 2 years later C.S.F. won the College World Series What Luck! at 19 I had my daughter She was So beautiful She is 8 Now. But at 19 ~~I killed many~~ I started doing ARMed Robberies and that was to keep my drug habbit up I Just didnt Care anymore. My last ARMed Robbery I took the police on a 55 Minute Police Chase through 3 freeways all the way to San on ofre powerplants. That was a crazy time in my life. I was fighting 15 years to life at 19 years old and had only Spent a couple of days in Jail Before that. It was a turn around. Eventually they dropped it down to a 4 year 4 Month Stay of Sentence with a Strike and a Release to a program. I graduated the program But was Still using I did a crime that involved Buying Flat Screen tv's with Fake money and returning them to get all real money Back. The FBI When I got arrested later Came and Interviewed me. But During This time while I was doing all that I really took my love for music to A New Height And after Stopping Sports altogether I went Fulltime Into music. I loved my guitar my piano and loved to write music I came into Contact With the right people and put out a Demo Cd for acoustic music and played a few Cool Coffee Shops. Somewher along The way I got asked If I would play Synthesiser IN a Band Called "Winds of Plague" So I did. This Really enhanced my drug use which was a large part of my downfall. I'll tell you this there is No Better drug then the feeling of Being on Stage Playing the music that you created In front of people. I should have Stuck with that. Instead of using Substances. I was weak and an idiot for being so weak for drugs. I continued music and Started

4

a Band called "Seconds from disaster" in which I sang. I played a lot of cool shows at a lot of cool places but Ruined all of that for drugs. Their is nothing glorious about drugs you Better be expecting to live in the darkest places and go through the worst of everything if you use drugs Eventually that outcome will come. Well Before I knew it I was on the Run and having Just committed new crimes I came home to my studio apartment and it was torn up the US Marshalls had found me I turned around to Run and Next thing I Know I had 8 Red dots on my chest. I was on my way to prison. After I lost my scholarship my dad wanted nothing to do with me so I was in this alone. That was 2011.

I've Been IN PRISON NOW for 4 years I really hadnt learned any lesson In the 1st 3 years I was in prison And ENded up Catching a case For drug paraplenilia while IN prison. So Now altogether I will do close to 6 years due to my drug use. Due to drugs I have Maxed out 2 terms Now And gotten in plenty of fights and lost plenty of friends & loved ones Along the way. Something clicked IN me after my 3rd year I realize I need to do Better I have people that need me and love me out there And By the time I get out my daughter Will Be 10 It's Not Fair to her at all I'm better then this And Prison is not Cool. Come here if you like violence, living in small spaces, Being told When you can eat, when you can shower, when you can go outside, and where you can sit. Racial violence is very high and you never know when things Can get ugly. All you have to do to stay out is do the Right thing and stay Sober. Don't try to be cool or be Someone your not. Just Do the Right thing. For My self I am gonna try to do the Right thing Be a Better PERSON Not

Just for me but for my daughter. I wasted so much of my life Now. I am capable of Reaching the Stars and I wont Stop till I do.

X My Name is Lance Thomas. And I give you Consent to use this however you See fit.

X Lance Thomas     10/16/14
Lance Thomas

I've been in prison now for four years. I really didn't learn any lesson in the first three years in prison, and ended up catching a case for drug paraphernalia while in prison. Altogether I will do close to six years—I'm currently only twenty-six years old. I have maxed out two terms now and gotten in plenty of fights and lost plenty of friends and loved ones along the way.

Something clicked with me after my third year, and I realized I needed to do better. I have people who need me and love me on the outside, and by the time I get out, my daughter will be ten years old.

Prison is not cool. Come here if you like violence, living in small spaces, and being told when you can eat, when you can shower, when you can go outside, and where you can sit.

All you have to do to stay out, is do the right thing; and stay sober, and stay clean. Don't try to be cool or be someone you're not. Just do the right thing.

One phrase from so many who have told or shared their stories rings true every time I read it: "Don't do it." The ride is not worth the cost. Often, the cost to start is free, but what follows is anything but free.

You will pay with your life, in one way, or another.

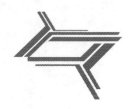

# WHERE DID THEY
# MOVE MY CHEESE?

Have you read the book *Who Moved My Cheese?* by Spencer Johnson? The "cheese" in Johnson's story is a metaphor for whatever it is we desire most in life—recognition, acceptance, money, relationships, possessions, freedom, or anything tangible or intangible.

In Spencer' story, mice are placed on one end of a maze, and cheese, their source of survival, is placed at the other end. As the mice begin their search for food, most will adapt quickly and find their cheese easily. Some, however, have a more difficult time locating their cheese.

At the heart of the book is the assertion, "Old beliefs do not lead you to new cheese." Individuals who are most open to the possibilities of change will fare well; others believe change will harm them, therefore resisting it. The problem with our world is that cheese is portable, leaving a person to navigate a mazelike world in a somewhat desperate search for fulfillment and satisfaction.

For the mice in the maze, after several weeks of the cheese being in the same place, it is relocated to another area. The mice are forced to begin a new mission to locate their cheese. Some, using their natural senses, locate their cheese quite easily, while others spend hours going in circles before locating their cheese. Still, a few will simply return to the original location and give up. They die because they cannot locate their cheese; they are creatures of habit, lacking the ability to survive or adjust to change.

People with addictions are similar creatures of habit. They check into a treatment program where they gain access to classes and various treatments, including medication, to help with detox and sustained sobriety. Thirty days, sixty days, or ninety days is a typical length of time for most, but when their program ends, they are again released to the world from which they came, on their own—but their cheese has been relocated.

Some will transition well, while others will waver back and forth before locating their cheese. Sadly, some will simply walk in circles before returning to the original location in search of their cheese (or their life-support system). A few will die because they relapse; a few will die because they cannot survive without their new "life-support system"; and others simply give up—the search is too daunting, the change too overwhelming. It's back to square one on how to survive in the very world in which they failed to navigate.

You can run in circles, hide in new places, or stow away in new surroundings, but you're still the same person when you look in the mirror. For sobriety to work, change needs to come from within, as well as your surroundings and the company you keep.

Many young adults in treatment had barely learned to survive on their own (given their age bracket, sixteen to twenty-two) before they ventured into the world of addiction. Upon completion of their program, the door is once again opened, and they reenter the world, but their cheese (their family, friends, source of survival) has been moved. Do we teach them to navigate to a new location, or do we leave them to struggle, yet again, on their own?

I choose to continue teaching my son how to manage his life, cautious to the fact that the road is a little more challenging and his task has a greater risk. I will lead him to the cheese many times before I feel secure in leaving him on his own. I will not enable him; I will simply help him navigate the maze. I will not move the cheese without showing him how to find it.

The road to recovery and continued sobriety doesn't end when a treatment program is over; it actually starts, when the door to freedom reopens.

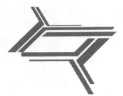

# WHAT I'VE LEARNED IN
# FOUR AND A HALF YEARS

I t is hard to believe; it has been four and a half years—1,602 days, to be exact—since first I learned of my son's disease, his addiction to drugs. Sadly, there is nothing else in my life that I count in days. I'll bet if I put my mind to the task, I could also calculate that number into the hours, minutes, and seconds that have passed since that dreadful day in February 2010. It's been 38,448 hours, or 2,306,880 minutes, or 1,384,412,800 seconds of my life spent in fear. That's 1,384,412,800 seconds of my life that I will never get back—and I continue to count.

Some might say that's a woeful way to live my life, that I should live in the moment—and so I do. I live every moment as though it were the last time I might see, feel, or talk to my son. Addiction does that. Addiction turns lives upside down, and inside out, and it never looks back. Addiction has an agenda. Some of the greatest minds known to man have tried to stop this disease—yet here we are, still counting.

So what have I learned in those 1,384,412,800 seconds? Far too much and not nearly enough. I have learned:

1. No matter how much I may want it, I cannot stop addiction from hurting my child.
2. No matter how much I want it, I cannot stop my child from harming himself.
3. I am not in control of the outcome that addiction brings to the table.

4. If my child dies tomorrow, there are many who will judge me for my son's actions, for my son's disease.
5. When I text the people who can save my child; there is seldom a response from the person on the receiving end of my text message.
6. No matter how great my prayers are or how much I try to barter with God, there is no guarantee that my prayers will be answered—at least not the way I want them to be answered.
7. I am only as strong as my weakest moment.
8. I may jump in front of a speeding bullet, but the bullet will not penetrate me when it was meant for my child.
9. With each new relapse, the spiral down grows stronger and stronger and with greater intensity.
10. For my child, it takes only six weeks to go from clean and focused to depressed, and standing on the ledge, ready to jump.

I also have learned that I don't want to learn anymore, yet I am still surprised as to what I have yet to learn about the disease of addiction. While I am not surprised by the lack of genuine concern from those around me, I am still deeply concerned that there is no better system in place today than there was twenty years ago. We simply have more facilities capitalizing on the desperate need, for more facilities. Don't get me wrong—for many facilities' the main goal is to help those in need to find their way back, however, the problem is, they are few and far between and not always available when a crisis arises.

What I've learned in four and a half years is just the tip of the iceberg when it comes to addiction. What I have learned in four and a half years is not nearly enough to save my child. What I have learned in four and a half years is not nearly enough … but it is all I have.

My prayers today are rather simple in comparison to those of my youthful prayers. I no longer ask for a million dollars or for the best and biggest Christmas gift. I no longer pray that my high school sweetheart will notice me. I no longer pray that my brothers will stop teasing me. Today, I simply whisper through my tears:

Dear Lord, in the next 1,384,412,800 seconds of my life, please change the way we treat those who suffer from the disease of addiction. And dear Lord, please help us to save more lives than we stand to lose over the next 1,384,412,800 seconds.

If you can live your life and bring happiness to someone in need, then your life has purpose. Far too many look at their life and ask "why me?" or "why not me?" A select few will look at their life and say, "Allow me," or "Let me." Which one are you?

It isn't easy to offer assistance to someone in need when you are in need as well. It isn't easy to say, "Allow me," when you want to say, "Help me." If we are not here to offer help to those less fortunate, then we are alone in our being. Our life will offer little value if we isolate from those around us.

There is always a reason to smile; there is always a reason to say thank you, just as there is a reason to say, "You're welcome," especially when a thank-you has been extended to you.

I would like thank all who bravely shared their journey or shared the story of a precious loved one gone too soon. Maybe nothing in this world can begin to ease the pain of such a loss, but I have a profound hope that in telling your story, someone else may find the strength to say, "I need help." Perhaps your story of survival or the story shared about a loved one's struggles will be a safety net for someone seeking help.

For all who have lost a loved one to this terrible disease, here is my message that I hope will bring you a small measure of comfort:

"If the essence of my being causes you to smile, or brings a brief moment of peace, then my mission in life was worth the journey."

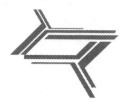

# MEDITATIVE SECTION

**Thoughts to Provoke Meditation**

In this section of *Parallel Worlds*, I offer some inspirational and thought thought-provoking observations. As you consider each phrase, allow your mind to settle on the meaning that follows, and then allow your mind to gently add your own thoughts or interpretations. As you wander back to this section of the book from time to time, I hope you find comfort in reading your own meditative expressions.

**Dream like there's no tomorrow.**
We all need dreams and goals and fantasies, but we also need to find ways to turn some of our dreams into realities. If you dream your life away, you may be left with *only* a dream at the end of the day.

_____

_____

_____

_____

**"If" is the middle word in "life."**
Is it just a coincidence that the word "if" is the middle word in Life? I don't think so.

_____

_____

_____

_____

**Smile every day until it feels natural.**
I try to smile every single morning when I rise; it sets the tone for the day. Some days are more difficult than others, and those are the days when I need to smile the most. Life is not always a bed of roses—and even roses have thorns. So smile at the simple things that life hands you.

_____

_____

_____

_____

**What is your "aha" moment?**
Do you know what an "aha" moment is? It's when you see something, feel something, or do something so special that all you can say is "Aha!" What is your aha moment?

_____

_____

_____

_____

**Allow your head to follow your heart.**
Sometimes we over-analyze a situation by allowing our mind to do all the thinking. Allow your heart a chance to lead the way. You might be inspired by where it leads you.

_____

_____

_____

_____

**I win—I love you.**
A simple game my daughter and I play is to see who will be the first one to say, "I win—I love you." Play your own game and see what happens. This one makes me smile every time we play.

_____

_____

_____

_____

**Even if you reach the top, you still have to climb over!**
Many people strive to achieve _one_ big goal in life and then stop. If you climb over and start the next goal in your life, you'll keep on living your dream.

_____

_____

_____

_____

**Remember musical chairs? When the music stops, the best position to be in just might be the one left standing.**

When the music stops, and you're the one left standing without a chair, you might think the game is over. However, you now have a chance to move on to the next game, while everyone else continues to walk in circles, waiting for the game to end. You are now in the perfect position to be first in line for the next game.

_____

_____

_____

_____

**Skating over thin ice doesn't necessarily make you brave.**

Sometimes in life, we take chances—and that can be a good thing. But taking too many chances can be a dangerous way to live your life. Sometimes, the bravest people are those who think before jumping off the cliff. Make sure you take the time to see if there is a safety net below.

_____

_____

_____

_____

**Not all decisions are set in stone.**
If you make a decision that turns out to be the wrong decision or not the best decision, you can usually find a way to change it. That doesn't mean you should change every decision you make; it simply means, not all decisions have to be a final decision.

_____

_____

_____

_____

**The fire can't burn if you don't strike the match.**
Sitting back and watching your life pass by is like watching the parade. If you have a plan, then strike the match and let the fire catch on.

_____

_____

_____

_____

**What does it take to win the gold?**
Olympic athletes spend years perfecting their skill before attempting to win the gold medal. Only a handful will take home the gold. Those who lose will spend another four years practicing, before trying again. So what are you waiting for? Start practicing.

_____

_____

_____

_____

**If you want to win, try nominating yourself.**
Don't wait around for someone to hand you the prize or pat you on the back; be your own hero, make your own movie, and set your own stage. Nominate yourself, and allow yourself to feel good about what you've accomplished.

_____

_____

_____

_____

**Somewhere in the middle is just fine.**
Most people want to be in the front of the line or the last one picked as a volunteer for a new job. I prefer to be somewhere in middle. Somehow, I always come out the winner. I don't have to start the ball rolling, and I don't have to worry too much about how the story ends.

_____

_____

_____

_____

**I'll take two No. 1's and a side of fries, please.**
Wouldn't it be easier if you could order your life the way you order your food? It's all spelled out for you; you just have select by number. You add side dishes or special-order your burger. Life is a bit more complicated, but then again, there are menu selections. You just have to know where to find them.

_____

_____

_____

_____

**Whatever!**
Do you ever have a day when no matter how hard you try, it's just not going to come together? Those are my "whatever" days. You can't spend too much time trying to figure them out; you just have to go with the flow.

_____

_____

_____

_____

**Every relationship needs a flower and a gardener.**
Which came first—the flower or the gardener? I don't know for sure, but without both, you have nothing. Relationships are similar; someone gets to be the flower, and someone has to tend the garden. It's a win/win situation, as long as you don't forget to take turns.

_____

_____

_____

_____

**It's not what helps you sleep at night; it's what keeps you awake!**
You can take a pill to fall asleep, but it might be better to find out what is keeping you awake. Turning off the day's problems isn't as simple as turning off the lights.

_____

_____

_____

_____

**If life is full of stepping stones, then why are my feet always wet?**
People often say that we have a path to follow. Is that path your stepping stone? You may need to get your feet wet from time to time in order to find the right stepping stones to support your life or your path.

_____

_____

_____

_____

**Don't stop too long on the path. Grass may start to grow.**
You should take the time to stop and smell the flowers—just don't pause too long. It may be difficult to start up again.

_____

_____

_____

_____

**Never regret anything that makes you smile.**
I'm not talking about smiling or laughing at the expense of someone else's feelings, but if you find yourself smiling when you see or hear something funny, then smile big and laugh out loud. Life is full of serious moments, but it's the little things we hold near and dear to our heart, that can make us smile.

_____

_____

_____

_____

**Life may not be the party you'd hoped for, but while you're here, you might as well dance.**
Not everything in life turns out the way you'd hoped it would. Just be willing to dance when you hear the music. Your life just might be someone else's inspiration.

_____

_____

_____

_____

**Starting a new tomorrow can't happen until today ends.**
Some days are just meant to be over. If you're having one of "those" days, just go with the flow, try to make the best of it, and then rest and wait for a new tomorrow.

_____

_____

_____

_____

**Dream of the impossible; reach for the probable.**
Dream big and dream outside the box, but don't be disillusioned if the dream is different than you'd planned. Always reach for the stars, but remember to look at what lies in front of you. It might be a dream begging to be recognized.

_____

_____

_____

_____

**Laugh out loud, even if no one hears you. Your heart will hear.**
I love laughing out loud. Sometimes people stop to see what I'm laughing at and then find themselves laughing along with me—and they don't even know why. Laughter is the best medicine; it makes your heart skip a beat. My heart always remembers the things that made me laugh.

_____

_____

_____

_____

**If you find yourself stumbling, try a route with fewer speed bumps.**
If you keep stumbling day after day, you might be on the wrong path.
Try the path less traveled. Maybe the job is not for you, or perhaps the
relationship is too much work. If things in your life aren't working, maybe
it's time to find a new route.

_____

_____

_____

_____

**The stars shine even in daylight. You just have to try harder to see them.**
Not everything in life is black or white. You may have to look a little
deeper to find your answers, but they're usually out there. Try a different
approach. Step back, take a second look, and ask for someone else's
opinion.

_____

_____

_____

_____

**If you hold someone's hand gently and tug a little less, he or she may be more willing to follow.**

You don't always have to be the leader; it can be an exhausting job. Pushing your way through the line only gets you in the door; it may not take you to the finish line.

_____

_____

_____

_____

**The longer the bridge, the more supports needed.**

If you have a big decision to make, you may need the support of family and friends. All bridges need support in order to hold the weight. Make sure your bridge has the support it needs.

_____

_____

_____

_____

**Even the smallest wave makes it to the shore eventually.**
The best-laid plans often start with little ideas. Little ideas can turn into big dreams, and big dreams are what keep us going. Start small and work your way up. You'll make it to the shore eventually, even if you need to use the tide to carry you the rest of the way home.

_____

_____

_____

_____

**Practice may make perfect, but persistence pays off every time.**
You can practice something over and over again and still not be good at it, but being persistent is entirely different. Make your thoughts known. Be the one people see the most often—strive to be seen. The outcome may be the greatest reward ever.

_____

_____

_____

_____

**Wash your hair, brush your teeth, clean your face. What cleanses your soul?**

Your outward appearance is usually well tended, but what do you do at the end of the day to cleanse your soul? Some people use prayers, some use meditation, and others simply turn off the lights.

---

---

---

---

**Jogging may get you there faster, but you might miss the journey along the way.**

Every day is a rush to the finish line—rush to get to work, rush to get home, rush the kids into bed, rush to watch a little TV before the day is over. Don't miss the journey in life. You only get one chance each day— use it wisely.

---

---

---

---

**Babies laugh for no apparent reason.**
Don't you wish you could just laugh for no apparent reason? Try it today, and see if it makes a difference. It may be a little difficult at first, but practice makes perfect! Now go out and find something that makes you laugh. *Find your inner baby.*

_____

_____

_____

_____

**You may not smile when it's raining, but you can still laugh when you jump in the puddles.**
Everyone has a bad day now and then—it's raining and you're running late for work or to get the kids to school. Perhaps it's time to stop for five minutes and jump in the puddle. Find a way to laugh at the gray clouds. They too will pass.

_____

_____

_____

_____

**If you keep stretching, you're bound to reach the stars.**
It's only when you stop searching for the next rainbow that you fail to notice the rainbow in front of you. Jump into each day with two feet. It will make you more stable.

_____

_____

_____

_____

**It only hurts when I'm breathing, but stopping isn't an option.**
Sometimes you lose your way, and you begin to slow down, almost as though you've stopped breathing. It may be time to look for something to remind you to take a deep, deep breath and jump back into the game.

_____

_____

_____

_____

**Hey diddle-diddle, the cat and the fiddle.**
That nursery rhyme makes me smile every time I say it. Find your own fun phrase. There are lots of them out there. "Hey diddle-diddle" is my happy fiddle. What's yours?

_____

_____

_____

_____

**Is it difficult living under a microscope?**

You are your own worst enemy. Every time you find fault with your personality, or your looks, or your job, it's like putting yourself under a microscope. Everyone gets to look at the cells and pull them apart. Stop looking so deeply, and start enjoying what's right in front of you.

_____

_____

_____

_____

**At one point, crumbs were part of the bigger picture.**

If you drop a cookie, it crumbles into pieces, but at one time, each piece was part of the whole picture. If you pull apart every aspect of your life, you might lose the bigger picture and be left with only the crumbs. Don't settle for the crumbs. Put all the pieces back together, and start building a bigger cookie.

_____

_____

_____

_____

**When a flower loses all its petals, is it still a flower?**

He loves me; he loves me not. Most of us played this game when we were children, but I was always afraid I would be left with no petals when I reached "he loves me not." Now, I play the game a little differently. He loves me, I love him back, they love me, and I love them too. Either way you look at it, someone is being loved. Works for me!

_____

_____

_____

_____

**Finish the play; then go home and relax.**

At the end of the day you need to find a way to get past the day's work, and go home and relax. Don't bring your day into your evening. Go home tonight, wipe your feet at the door, and brush off the stress of the day. Then walk in and smile—this is your time to relax.

_____

_____

_____

_____

**Is a balloon still a balloon without hot air?**
So many things in life are defined by what we put into them. Balloons are still balloons, with or without your hot air. They look better when inflated, though, so inflate your life. The more you put into it, the more you'll get out of it.

_____

_____

_____

_____

**A house of glass is better than a heart of glass.**
With a house of glass, people can see what's inside. You need not hide from who you are, but if your heart is made of glass, you will need to hold it so tightly to keep it from shattering. What kind of heart do you want? If your heart is open and warm, it's easier to feed.

_____

_____

_____

_____

**When was the last time you skipped rocks on the water?**
Kids find it so easy to just be kids. Why is it that when we become adults, we think we must to stop having fun? Try skipping rocks, and it won't be long before you remember how to smile. It will be contagious.

_____

_____

_____

_____

**I just decided that I will no longer dwell on it.**
If you dwell on a problem, does it really go away? Not every problem is solved by over-thinking it. Sometimes you just have to let go to find the solution.

_____

_____

_____

_____

**If I ran the world ...**
Take the time to write your own future. If you could run the world, what would you do? If you could change your life, what would you change? Change is fun; change is good; change keeps you alive and in the game.

_____

_____

_____

_____

**Feed your imagination.**
Every day is a new day to imagine a new beginning, create a new strategy, or a find new solution to an old problem. Let today be the day you imagine your new future. Let today be the day to imagine a new beginning. Feed your imagination.

---

**Let the simple things become the important things.**
Sometimes the simple things in life are the important things in our memory. Don't try to make everything you do so big that you lose out on the fun in getting there. Keep it simple, keep it light, and keep it little. The simple things in life often become everlasting memories in your heart.

---

**Babies don't care if you're rich or poor.**
You don't have to prove yourself to be the hero in a baby's eye. Somewhere along the way, many of us decide we need to be bigger than life to be loved. This could not be farther from the truth. We are loved for who we are, not for what we have.

_____

_____

_____

_____

**Don't circumvent the middle.**
The middle of the book is the good stuff, and so is the middle of your life. If you try to sidestep the middle, you'll get to the end way too quickly. I'd rather savor the middle, think about the beginning, and plan for the future. Doughnuts are the only things in life that are better without the middle.

_____

_____

_____

_____

**Don't worry so much about what you're feeling today. By the time you figure it all out, it's already changed.**

Some days are better left alone. You've changed your mind today more times than you've changed your outfit, and maybe that's okay. If you're feeling out of sorts today, then just go with the flow and allow the silence to lead you in a new direction.

---

---

---

---

**If you turn right four times, do you end up back where you started?**

Some days you just find yourself going in circles. These are the days when you're probably better off making fewer right turns. Maybe you need to take a step back in order to clear the path for a new direction.

---

---

---

---

**When did okay become okay?**

Seventy percent will get you through to the next grade, and 70 percent will probably be okay to finish up your daily job, but is it really all you want for your life? Okay is okay, but you can do better. You may not always need to finish with 100 percent to be successful, but always strive for better than "okay."

_____

_____

_____

_____

**You can't get to the shore without riding the waves.**

No one gets to the shore without riding a wave, even a small wave. Many situations in life are similar to waves in the ocean. There are big waves, and there are small waves in everything we do—the people we turn to when we need help and the people we help when they are in need. Waves are all around. Catch one, and find out where it takes you.

_____

_____

_____

_____

**Why is four out of five okay, and why can't we get number five onboard?**
Do those commercials bother you, where you're told "four out of five" experts agree on something? They bother me. Everyone is on board with the plan except number five. Then again, it goes to show you that you can't please everyone, so stop trying. If you get four out of five on your side, you're doing just fine.

---

---

---

---

**I'm logging off now!**
I wish I were a computer. When I get too tired, someone will turn me off and let me rest. I think today when I've had enough, I'll just send everyone I know a message: "I'm logging off now." I wonder if they'll get it.

---

---

---

---

**If there were no tomorrow, would today still exist?**
Are you putting off your happiness because you think tomorrow will be better? What if there were no tomorrow? What a waste of today.

---

---

---

---

**I'll take two "E" tickets, please.**
At one time, an entrance package at Disneyland was made up of "A," "B," and "C" tickets, but the most popular of all was the "E" ticket. E tickets were reserved for the best rides in the park, and each booklet of tickets contained four or five E tickets; those were saved for the end of the evening. Life is similar in many ways. You work your entire life, saving your free time to enjoy the E-ticket ride. What if life ended before you got to enjoy the E ticket?

_____

_____

_____

_____

**When you think you've reached the bottom, look for a loophole.**
There's always a loophole. Lawyers use them all the time as a way out of a situation. Life has loopholes, though they usually come in forms not easily recognized. You may have to dig a little deeper, but they're out there. Now go find your loophole.

_____

_____

_____

_____

**Before you embark on a journey of revenge, dig two graves.**
No one is the winner when revenge is part of the game. Everyone loses. Rather than seeking revenge, seek knowledge. Try to find a better way to understand the situation. Revenge has no winners.

---

**Never make an enemy out of a lawyer.**
This is almost too much of a cliché to even dive into, but here goes. There are know-it-alls in every game. Use your common sense to distinguish good advice from bad.

---

**You don't need to know all the words in order to sing the song.**
If you're sitting on the sidelines waiting for your chance to join in the fun, you may be there for a very long time. If you know the chorus, then sing the chorus, and hum your way through the rest of the song. Life is similar. There's a beginning, a middle, and an end. Jump in before the song is over.

---

**What you see depends on what you're looking for.**
How many times was there a rainbow in the sky, but you forgot to notice? Every day is a chance to notice what's right in front of you. If you like what you see, then cherish it. If you don't like what you see, then change it. Change directions, change attitudes, or change your mind, but always notice a rainbow.

_____

_____

_____

_____

**If you give up, your dream may not become reality.**
There are many things that are not worth the time spent to think about them. But there are many times when we give up before it becomes a reality. If you give up too quickly, your dream won't have time to turn into something worth keeping.

_____

_____

_____

_____

**Is the impact of your past directing your future?**
There's a reason why it's called the past. The past can be a fun place to visit from time to time, but if you spend your life there, you may run out of time for a future.

_____

_____

_____

_____

**Today, I'll make friends with myself.**
The best place to start is by looking in the mirror, not to see what you look like on the outside but to talk to the person on the inside. Have a conversation with yourself. If you fall asleep in the middle, chances are, you need to reinvent you!

_____

_____

_____

_____

**If you spend all day looking for motivation, you may run out of time to be motivated.**

Motivation is great; we all need it, but don't sit around all day telling yourself, "I'm looking for something or someone to motivate me." Eight hours will pass, and you'll still be sitting there. Try waking up and telling yourself, "The first thing I see when I open the door will be my inspiration for the day." You'll find yourself thinking outside the box as you look for something new to motivate you.

_____

_____

_____

_____

**You can fly around all day; just don't forget to land.**

Jumping into life with two feet is great, and so is flying from one project to the next. But if you don't plant your feet on the ground from time to time, you'll never enjoy the fruits of your own labor.

_____

_____

_____

_____

**Is the music inside my head bothering you?**

We all dance to the music in our heads at some point, but if your music bothers everyone around you, you might want to change the channel. That doesn't mean you need to conform to the needs of everyone else, but maybe you just need to listen to someone else's music every once in a while.

---

---

---

---

**My GPS system isn't working.**

Have you ever had one of those days when all you wanted to do was stop? If you turn off your GPS system, maybe you can do just that. Relax, and pull off the road for a minute or two. The GPS system may tell you where you're going, but sometimes you have to pull off the road and reset your compass.

---

---

---

---

**Where is the purple in my sunset?**

I love to watch the sunset until the purple shows through. It's the prettiest part of the transformation. Far too many people see a sunset and say, "Oh, how pretty," and then turn and walk away. Try watching until the end, and see what happens.

_____

_____

_____

_____

**The battle began long before the first bullet left the gun.**

You might think the battle started when the first shot was fired, but it started long before that. Anger builds up, words are tossed out, and without further warning, the battle is set in motion. The next time anger starts to build up, extinguish it before the bullet can leave the gun. You might just prevent the war.

_____

_____

_____

_____

**The stop sign isn't the end; it's just a momentary pause.**
When you come to a stopping place in life, pause for a gentle moment to regroup, and then proceed to the next stop sign. Each pause is a resting place that prepares you for the journey ahead. Life is all about enjoying the pauses.

_____

_____

_____

_____

**"Twinkle Twinkle Little Star" is more than just a song.**
Childhood songs are great, but many people believe they are only for kids. I love to sing a little-kid song when I'm in a good mood or at a crossroad in my life. They make me smile, and they make me think with a clearer vision. Try it, and see where it takes you. It may result in nothing more than a smile, but hey, a smile can be great.

_____

_____

_____

_____

**Make your own puzzle pieces.**
I loved puzzles when I was a kid. There were so many pieces to find, and I was always so delighted when all the pieces fell into place. What a great picture I just created. As a grown-up, I like to make my own puzzle pieces. I like to be surprised at what is right in front of me, once I've designed my own puzzle.

---

---

---

---

**Anyone can throw the first punch.**
Every fight starts with a punch—maybe a physical one, maybe a verbal one, but either way, someone has to "punch" first. Why not try something different today? Step back, smile, and say, "No thanks. I think I'll just sit this one out." It may not end the argument, but it may cause someone else to reconsider joining it.

---

---

---

---

**Walk in step to your own music.**

It's easier to walk in step to someone else's music than it is to make up your own. But in the long run, walking in step to your own music or walking on your own path is much more rewarding.

_____

_____

_____

_____

**If we are all heroes, then there's no one left to applaud as we walk by.**

I like to be noticed as an important person in a meeting, and I enjoy the accolades that come with winning the game, but sometimes it's nice to side on the curb and applaud someone else's accomplishments. Let someone else enjoy being the hero today.

_____

_____

_____

_____

**You could be right all the time, but why would you want to be?**

Some people love being right all the time, but why? It's very exhausting.

_____

_____

_____

_____

**Sometimes, no news is good news.**
If you're waiting for all the answers to life's questions to come in a neatly packaged box, you'll have a long wait. Sometimes the things you believe you want most are the very things you need least in your life. Sometimes there are no answers, and it's okay to move on to a new project. Sometimes no news is the answer.

_____

_____

_____

_____

**Let go long enough to start over.**
Holding on to all the old stuff doesn't leave much room for the new stuff. It takes a lot to understand the difference between letting go of something and holding on to something that is no longer working. Maybe the best stuff is yet to come.

_____

_____

_____

_____

**Sometimes the pieces fit better after you break them apart.**
A puzzle may start out as a whole picture, but it becomes a puzzle once it's broken apart. The fun is in finding how the pieces fit together. Life is similar. Sometimes you need to break apart all the pieces in order to find the whole picture again.

_____

_____

_____

_____

**In some games, it's the handicap that counts.**
In golf, the handicap is important and is not considered a "handicap" by definition. Many areas of our lives require us to complete a task with minimal attempts. Sometimes restrictions are put in place to help us complete our mission in a timely manner.

_____

_____

_____

_____

**Broken dreams are still dreams; they just have more pieces.**
If your dream becomes a broken dream, you might attempt to toss it out and start over—but maybe you shouldn't. Maybe all you need is to look at your dream in a different way. It's still a dream, but maybe it will have a different outcome.

_____

_____

_____

_____

**Not every memory deserves a permanent place in your mind.**
Memories are moments in time reserved in our minds. If a memory is unpleasant, however, then toss it out and reserve the open space in your mind for more pleasant journeys.

_____

_____

_____

_____

**Not everything in life should be sugar-coated.**
Some problems just need to be tackled head-on. No sugar-coating will make them taste better. You may want to "sugar-coat" it to soften the blow, but chances are, the end result will be the same. Some things just need to be handled so you can move on to more important matters.

_____

_____

_____

_____

**Power isn't power when it becomes common.**
Exerting too much power all the time not only becomes boring, but it becomes common. People eventually stop listening. They'll turn away and look elsewhere for their information. Here's to a less powerful, uncommon day!

_____

_____

_____

_____

**Don't forget to drain the sink so you can fill it with fresh water.**
If you keep your mind filled with dirty water, then the clean water has no place to go. Stop dwelling on the things you cannot change. Clean them up as best you can, and move on.

_____

_____

_____

_____

**Does drinking Kool-Aid make you cool?**
How many times in life did we think we were cool because we followed in the footsteps of the "cool guy"? The "cool guy" might have more problems than you do; he just looks cooler while making an idiot out of himself. If you follow your own footsteps in life, you'll be cool enough.

_____

_____

_____

_____

**I'd love to start over. I just forget where the beginning is.**
Not all projects are meant to be finished. Some are just learning steps to greater things to come.

_____

_____

_____

_____

**I'm sorry—what were you saying?**
If your mind is no longer listening to what's being said around you, this might be a clue that it's time for a "time-out." Take a step back, inhale, exhale, and listen to a new CD.

_____

_____

_____

_____

**I've listened for so long that I've actually forgotten what we were talking about.**
Sitting on the sidelines is great. Letting someone else have the floor is also great. Just don't forget to jump back into the game every now and then. Some people are born to follow, but we all have a leader inside us, just waiting to be realized.

_____

_____

_____

_____

**Do you have a business card? I'd love to Google you.**
It seems like everyone has his or her name on a business card these days. Maybe they feel important when they hand the card to you, or maybe they have it to remind themselves of who they are. You can Google anything or anyone on the Internet, but half the fun of discovery is doing your own off-line research. Here's to a day without the computer.

_____

_____

_____

_____

**You may not like the bumps in the road, but without them, you'll never recognize the smooth road.**
It would be nice to imagine a day or a life without any speed bumps, but then again, if there were no bumps in the road, would your journey seem smoother? I'm not sure, but I believe the bumps in the road may help you to find a new direction.

_____

_____

_____

_____

**You could match power with power, but you'll never get anywhere.**
Being in charge or having power is exhilarating, but it can also be exhausting, especially when your power is matched with someone else's power. Look at each situation, and then decide whose power is more useful to complete the job at hand.

_____

_____

_____

_____

**Big waves require a tow-in.**
Big Wave Riders need to be towed in to the wave before they can surf it. Big problems in life may also require help or assistance or a tow-in. Success comes from all who help you achieve it. You don't have to do it alone all the time.

_____

_____

_____

_____

**Take two Chardonnays, and call me in the morning.**
Are you having one of "those" days? You can stop the merry-go-round
and climb off. All you have to do is hold up your hand and shout to the
conductor, "Hey, I need to get off this ride."

_____

_____

_____

_____

**I didn't know anything different, until I learned different**
What we know is what we've learned. We learn from our parents. We learn
from our friends, and we learn from our own life experiences. The real
question is, what will you teach yourself today?

_____

_____

_____

_____

**It doesn't matter who, what, or why—just find your own higher power.**
To whom we pray, to what we pray, or how we pray is not what's most important. What is important is that you acknowledge a higher power. Without one, you appoint yourself as your own higher power. You make yourself your own almighty, and you set yourself up for disappointment. You can't solve all of life's problems on your own. There are times when you need to let go and give your problems over to someone else—or something else. We all need someone or something greater than ourselves. Do you have a higher power?

_____

_____

_____

_____

**I'm always going to be perfectly imperfect.**
There is no such thing as perfection in oneself. We were not made to be perfect; we were made to be the best we can be. If you strive for perfection, you will surely disappoint yourself. Being the best "you" you can be is perfect enough. Strive for a better you.

_____

_____

_____

_____

**What is your "turn off" button?**

If you let each day roll into the next day, you may never achieve a completed task. You need to learn how to turn off yesterday, so you can start a fresh tomorrow. I can't imagine a day without a turn-off button. Today is a good day to find your own turn-off button.

_____

_____

_____

_____

**Terminal uniqueness—what a fun concept!**

We are terminally unique. Each of us has an opportunity to become unique in some way, shape, or form. What makes you stand out? What makes you different? What makes you tick? You are your own unique investment. Make today count.

_____

_____

_____

_____

**You don't complete me; you complement me.**
Have you ever heard the term, "You complete me"? I choose to believe I am complete all by myself. I do, however, like the idea that someone else can complement me. If you wait around for someone else to complete you, you may be waiting around forever. Find someone who complements you.

_____

_____

_____

_____

**Are you willing to change, or are you eager to change?**
With the right incentives, most people are "willing" to change or "willing" to try something new. However, those who are eager to change or to try something new will have done so for the right reasons. The only incentive you need to better yourself is the incentive—the eagerness—to expand your life.

_____

_____

_____

_____

**You have a right to have boundaries.**

You can set your own boundaries. You can say no to the things or people in your life that hold you back. You can change your direction by changing your boundaries. We all have boundaries; we just need to remind ourselves they exist.

_____

_____

_____

_____

**The "why" is not what matters.**

Don't spend so much time looking for the "why" in life. You will run out of time to live. Not everything we do requires a "why," nor can everything be explained. Be good to yourself, be kind to your heart, and be safe in your decisions. If you do this, there won't be a "why" in your life. There will just be a *life*.

_____

_____

_____

_____

**Normal is just a setting on your dryer.**
Think about this the next time you say, "I just want a normal day." For most people, a normal day is one with too much work, too much stress, and too little down time. Here's to an *abnormal* day—a day filled with relaxation, meditation, and the time to dream and think outside the box. *Normal is just a setting on your dryer.*

_____

_____

_____

_____

**Bottom-line it for me.**
It's nice to be pleasant and listen to every word that someone says, but sometimes you just have to get to the bottom line. If something in your life seems to be a never-ending battle, find a new way to get to the bottom line. There must be at least one solution you've yet to try.

_____

_____

_____

_____

**My lease on life is up. Where do I get a new one?**
We can lease a car, lease a condo, lease a house, lease furniture, lease appliances—and it appears we can lease a new life. I know this to be true, because I've heard it said, "I got a new lease on life." Now go out and find your new lease.

_____

_____

_____

_____

**Don't mind me; I'm just waiting to exhale.**
If you've been holding your breath for so long that you can't remember how to inhale deeply and exhale peacefully, it's time to take a break. Life can be exhilarating and exhausting at the same time, but that doesn't mean you can't call for a time-out—if for no other reason than to see if the game you started is still the game you're playing.

_____

_____

_____

_____

**If I sit with my eyes closed, will everyone think I'm gone?**

One more meeting, one more phone call, one more dinner to make, and one more load of laundry to finish—then I'm done. It would be nice if you could just make a list of the things you need to do, and when you're done writing it down, you're done! Finished! Close your eyes. No one can find you now. Try it. Make a list, finish your chores, and then close your eyes.

---

---

---

---

**God rested on the seventh day, and on the eighth day he said, "Okay, Murphy, you're in charge."**

Are you familiar with Murphy's Law? It's the idea that anything that can go wrong *will* go wrong. Does this relate to your life? If it doesn't, it probably will at some point. A variation of Murphy's Law is, "If there is a possibility of several things going wrong, the one that will cause the most damage will be the first one to go wrong." But this is true of most situations. If you plan to fail, you probably will. You could start your own version of Murphy's Law.

---

---

---

---

**If nothing is impossible why can't I dribble a football?**
I would love to think that nothing is impossible, but that's an unrealistic way to live my life. I'm a firm believer in trying to succeed in whatever I want, as long as I understand, that some things are just not meant to be. Maybe they're not impossible, but they're just not meant to be.

_____

_____

_____

_____

**Stop your limited-system thinking.**
What is limited-system thinking? It is the way in which we sabotage our own success by telling ourselves, "I can't do that," or "I'm not going to be able to understand that problem." Before you've even ventured into a new project, you've lined yourself up for failure when you start out with negative energy, negative thoughts, or negative patterns. Try thinking outside your own personal box, and give yourself permission to take a chance on something new. Give yourself the credit to own your success.

_____

_____

_____

_____

**God, if I can't have what I want, can I at least have what they have?**
Maybe what you want isn't really what you need. Wants and needs are different, and both come with conditions. If you want something badly enough, then find a way to accomplish your task. If you need something badly enough, find a way to earn it. Nothing in life comes without a price. Some things are purchased, and some things are earned. Make sure that what you want or what you need has value to you. Otherwise, you're just chasing someone else's dream.

_____

_____

_____

_____

**The voices in my head may not be real, but they do offer some interesting ideas.**
Thinking in detail about a plan can make all the difference in the outcome of the game. Talk to yourself. Have a conversation about your ideas and your plans before putting them into action. Let the voices in your head do some of the critical thinking.

_____

_____

_____

_____

**I'm often confused by my own actions.**

"Did I just do that? Hey, what am I doing here, and why did I think that was a good idea?" If your own actions confuse you, perhaps you are trying too hard or are trying to please everyone else. If you let your actions confuse you, the game will never be any fun.

_____

_____

_____

_____

**My mission in life is to lose responsibility.**

In this fast-paced, get-up, get-moving, conquer-the-world life we have made for ourselves, sometimes it's nice to lose or let go of some of our responsibilities. You don't have to conquer the world to be a responsible adult. You can let other people handle some projects. Try finding your balance. You may unearth a whole new world.

_____

_____

_____

_____

**Don't invite me onto the field if you're not going to let me play the game.**

We get invited into all types of situations, many of which have nothing to do with us. Do you find yourself wondering why you're here and what someone expects from you? Pay attention to how you participate in conversations; you may get invited into the game and still not be invited to play. Sometimes it's better to listen and acknowledge that you are present than to leave the rest of the game up to the other players.

_____

_____

_____

_____

**Are you fully participating in the creation of your own life?**

When you're old, tired, and ready to move on to the next life—heaven, hell, or somewhere in between—will you look back and say, "I created that life, and I lived it fully"? Or will you say, "That was a complete waste of time"? Don't wait too long to participate in your life. It will pass you by before you know it. Enjoy the ride, but change directions every now and then.

_____

_____

_____

_____

**Life isn't moving if you're peddling in place.**
Many people get up in the morning and follow the same routine, day in and day out. If it works, don't mess with it! But are you really getting anywhere, or are you peddling in place? Life seems good, so you don't rock the boat. If it isn't broke, don't fix it. These are familiar clichés. Remember to pedal to a new place every once in a while. If you don't, then you might miss the sunset on another island.

_____

_____

_____

_____

**Don't always look for like-minded people.**
It's often too easy to only seek people with similar interests or ideas. How can you learn new things if the conversation is no different from talking to yourself in the mirror? We need to welcome the opposition. The views may be different, but they may open your eyes to new possibilities.

_____

_____

_____

_____

**Everything in life is written between the lines.**
In life, you have to learn to read between the lines. Many ideas, opinions, or suggestions can be taken at face value, but many times the solution is somewhere in the middle. Sometimes you have to listen to the entire conversation, and then draw your own conclusion. Read the message in the middle before deciding on the outcome.

_____

_____

_____

_____

**Never curse the bad road that brings you to a good place.**
Life is full of choices and far too often, we make the poor choices. But if the choice you make bring you to a better place, then look at the choice as a learning curve. If you curse the initial choice and regret that you made it, you might not learn from the experience, and you'll stand a greater chance of making the same bad choice again.

_____

_____

_____

_____

**Don't include me in your mass text. I want to be special.**
Do you send mass e-mails, texts, or update letters to friends and family? Keep in mind that if your message says something special, or "I love you," the person who needs your message the most should be the only one receiving your message. If a friend or family member is in need of uplift, don't send words of encourage to that person—with a "CC" to everyone in your address book.

_____

_____

_____

_____

**Today, you tested clean.**
Sobriety is not easy, but it is possible. Today is the only day you have, and it's the only day that matters. Tomorrow has its own set of rules, and today is the first day you can take control. Today is the only day you can count on … so make it count.

_____

_____

_____

_____

**If you have no direction in life, then you'll never get where you thought you were going.**

You can get in your car or get on a plane a bus, but at some point you'll have to decide where you're going. It's your life and your choices. Some days are harder, and some days are easier, but all days require a direction.

_____

_____

_____

_____

**How long does it take to get to a hundred laughs?**

Today I laughed—once. Then I thought, *how long would to take for me to laugh one hundred times?* So I started counting—one day, two days, and fifteen days—and I didn't even get out of the starting gate. Make a purpose to laugh more today than yesterday. After a while, you'll find yourself laughing more than you thought possible. Laughter is good for the soul—and it's contagious!

_____

_____

_____

_____

**Artists paint pictures that change lives.**
Life is art, and art is life. If someone were to paint your life story, what would it say to the person admiring the painting? Think about it.

_____

_____

_____

_____

**Life is a potpourri of sanity.**
Life is not a simple task. No one gets out of it alive! There is so much for which to be thankful—just open your eyes and your heart to the possibilities. Change comes from everything you do, and how you see others. A rainbow is more than just a fleeting ray of hope in the sky—it's a reason to look up! And while you're looking up, find a reason to jump back into the game.

_____

_____

_____

_____

**Have you ever been on hold for so long that you've forgotten to whom you were talking?**

Every time you stop to think about your plan, it places your life on hold. I've sometimes sat for hours, even days, just trying to figure out where I'm going or what I'm doing. I've even gotten somewhere and then tried to remember why I wanted to go there in the first place. If thinking about your new plan puts you on hold, it might not be the right path or road, at least not for the moment. You can always revisit an old plan, but you can never get back lost time!

_____

_____

_____

_____

**Your apology is noted; my acceptance of it is pending.**
If someone apologizes for doing something or saying something that hurt your feelings, that doesn't mean you're obligated to accept the apology. You don't want to hold a grudge—that's a complete waste of time— but you can move past the situation without giving in. Make sure you understand the apology, and give your heart time to heal.

_____

_____

_____

_____

**This is your ticket back into the game.**

When you think you've lost your way, look for a sign to jump back into the game. Maybe a phone call will offer a solution, or maybe a friend will come from out of nowhere and serve as a guide. There is always a way back into the game, no matter how long you've been sitting on the sidelines.

_____

_____

_____

_____

**Live life as if you have a purpose.**

We all know that life is short, no matter how many years we have. Live your life with a purpose in mind. You wouldn't buy a house or car or plan an expensive trip without giving it a lot of thought, so why does your life require so little imagination? Life each day with a purpose in mind. Even if your plan for the day doesn't work out the way you'd hope it would, at least you gave it some thought.

_____

_____

_____

_____

**If your life were the script for a new reality show, would it be worth watching?**

How you live your life may reflect more than your personality. Someone might be looking to you for his or her answers. What type of reality show does your life represent?

_____

_____

_____

_____

**Bed bugs don't like dogs.**

I didn't know this was true until a recent "bed bug epidemic." But it did make me wonder what scent a dog gives out that protects it against bed bugs. Look around you, and see what type of mayhem your life is attracting. If you seem to be attracting negative energy, then change the "scent" of your personality. Don't let the bed bugs bite. Once they start, it's difficult to get rid of them.

_____

_____

_____

_____

**Pizza is like spinach for your brain.**
I love pizza. It may not be the healthiest food, but I do feel good when I eat it. Maybe spinach is better for us, but pizza makes the world go 'round. Find your own healthy version of pizza for your soul.

_____

_____

_____

_____

**Attitudes are contagious. Is yours worth catching?**
When someone around you has an unhealthy attitude, it is usually contagious. When you enter a room today, make sure your attitude is something worth showing or giving away.

_____

_____

_____

_____

**"Things go best for the people who make the best out of the way things turn out."**
**—John Wooden**

Making the best of a good situation is simple; making the best of a bad situation takes talent, and it takes courage. Make the best out of what you've been handed. Someone may be watching to see if you're worthy of the good stuff before they invest in your future.

_____

_____

_____

_____

**Success is only hindered by your fear of failure.**

We all want to be successful in our lives, and we all want to avoid making wrong choices, but if you avoid making choices out of fear of failure; you may wind up not making a choice at all. Failure is not always a bad thing; it may help you to better understand what good choices look like. Not too many people set their sights on poor choices. Use your best judgment, seek advice of others, and look for signs—they're out there!

_____

_____

_____

_____

**It's not what you do with the information you receive; it's what you don't do.**

Most every day we receive information via a telephone call, an e-mail, a tweet, or a Facebook post. Information helps us or hinders us, or it can uplift our souls.

_____

_____

_____

_____

**It's okay to be perfectly human.**

What is so wrong with being human? We are the same in so many ways, yet we strive to stand out, to be different. Being human means we can still be special, just not perfect.

_____

_____

_____

_____

**Are you reacting, or are you responding?**

When a situation arises, the manner in which you handle it will show others who you are. If you react harshly to something, you might be misunderstood or be seen as a person of hostility. If you respond to a situation calmly, you stand a better chance of getting your opinion heard.

---

---

---

---

**Now is the perfect time to fill in the blank spaces of your life. Start here, start simple, and start with a fresh perspective. Just start.**

_____

_____

_____

_____

_____

_____

_____

_____

_____

_____

_____

_____

_____

_____

_____

_____

_____

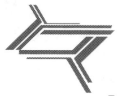

# IT STARTS WITH A SIMPLE
# CUP OF COFFEE

Have you ever sat in a coffeehouse and watched as people flocked in and out, endlessly for hours? All walks of life, all colors, all ages, all backgrounds—all together in one common place.

As I sat with a dear friend in a local coffeehouse, I couldn't help but wonder, *how did so many people with vastly different backgrounds all find their way to the same coffeehouse?* Could it be fate that brought so many to the same place? Could it actually be that a simple cup of coffee was the missing link to such a gathering—a gathering better known as the "common grounds" of life? Perhaps I am overthinking this concept, but maybe I'm on to something simple yet so profound that it may be the answer, to many unanswered questions.

If we could find a common ground for the things in life that alter our lives, perhaps we could find a way to work together toward a brighter tomorrow. There are countless people whose lives have been altered by things beyond their control, and there are many who will spend their entire life trying desperately to find a common ground upon which to live their life. Why is this such a difficult task to accomplish? Why are so many beautiful, young, and talented souls lost in a maze that was created for them, but not entirely, by them?

If only I had the answers—if only someone had the answers—for the common ground that could pull us together. We lose precious lives every single day, and many could have been saved; instead, they lost their battle as they fell into the abyss known as "stigma." What a terrible way to die—to die alone. To die afraid and lost, to die ashamed of a life lived. The disease of addiction has many wounded warriors, many casualties of the war, and many POWs.

Disease is described as a particular abnormal, pathological condition that affects part or all of an organism. In humans, the word "disease" often refers to any condition that causes pain, dysfunction, distress, social problems, or death to the person afflicted.

Disease usually affects people physically as well as emotionally, as contracting or living with many diseases, can alter one's perspective on life and greatly alter one's personality.

Death by disease is often referred to as "death by natural causes." I do not consider death by disease a "natural" cause, especially when the disease is highly treatable. There are different types of diseases, but in humans, perhaps the deadliest and most disturbing disease is the one that could have been prevented.

Heart disease, for example, may be caused by consumption of fatty foods, a sedentary lifestyle, or other unhealthy lifestyle choices; seldom does the life-altering stigma follow heart disease, as it does with the disease of addiction. Where is the praise and encouragement for those struggling with the disease of addiction? Where are the trained coaches? Where is the lifetime of assistance? Where is the safety net?

If the victim of the disease of addiction has an unending supply of money, perhaps they stand a chance to win the battle. But what happens to the thousands who beg for help but can't afford a viable treatment program? What happens in the desperate hours between detox and waiting for an open "free" spot in a treatment facility? Death is often the outcome.

What if *every* disease in which the victim somehow contributed to the onset of their disease, were treated the same across the board? What if *every* disease in which the victim had a choice—but made the wrong choice, faced the same consequences: incarceration, legal issues, or a lifetime of stigma? If this were the case, perhaps it would bring forth an environment of greater understanding, greater empathy, and less ignorant assumptions?

Yes, many diseases start with *one poor choice*. But the similarities often end there.

The disease of addiction carries—for those who survive—a life sentence of stigma. The word "addiction" resides in a class by itself.

Perhaps the deadliest disease in humans—is *the **disease of IGNORANCE.***

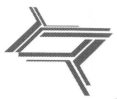

# For Now, My Journey Ends Here

I hope my story and the stories from those who contributed to *Parallel Worlds* will encourage you to open your heart to the greatest possibility: "There is hope, and there is a way to survive this journey."

Offer your heart and leave the stigma and judgment behind. Walk softly and leave a lasting impression for those who may follow.

If addiction has taken over the life of someone you love, you have three choices: You can let it destroy you, you can allow it to define you, or you can let it strengthen you. The final choice is up to you.

*Kathleen McGill*
*Mother, photographer, writer*

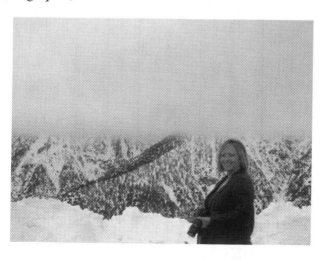